How to Safeguard
Your Health and Beauty
By the Simple Pressure
of a Finger

By the same author

How to Give Yourself Relief from Pain by the Simple Pressure of a Finger

How to Safeguard
Your Health and Beauty
By the Simple Pressure
of a Finger

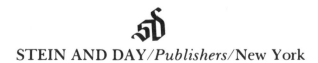

Dr. Roger Dalet

Translated by Linda Zuck

STEIN AND DAY/*Publishers*/New York

First published in the United States of America in 1983
Copyright © 1979 Opera Mundi, Paris
Translation © 1980 Hutchinson Publishing Group, London
Revised translation © 1983 Stein and Day/*Publishers*
All rights reserved, Stein and Day, Incorporated
Printed in the United States of America
Stein and Day/*Publishers*
Scarborough House
Briarcliff Manor, N.Y. 10510

Library of Congress Cataloging in Publication Data

Dalet, Roger.
    How to safeguard your health and beauty by the simple pressure of a
finger.

    Translation of Sauvegardez vous-même votre santé et votre beauté
par simple pression d'un doigt.
Includes index.
    1. Acupressure.   2.   Beauty, Personal. 3.   Health.
I. Title.
RM723.A27D3513   1983   615.8'22   80-5497
ISBN 0-8128-2742-2

Contents

Introduction

In the book *How to Give Yourself Relief from Pain by the Simple Pressure of a Finger,* we presented a method of obtaining rapid relief from everyday aches and pains using specific pressure points which, when stimulated, provide relief from discomfort.

This simple method, without recourse to drugs or chemical products of any kind, can also be used preventively, both to maintain and to restore the natural harmony of the body.

In other words, we are talking about *safeguarding* health.

Western medicine today is increasingly concerned with preventive care but is often not fully aware how best to achieve it. This book is a contribution to that end.

Health equals beauty

Health and beauty complement, and are conditional on, one another. If you doubt this, consider the following two examples. Safeguarding the beauty of the face means more than preserving the freshness of the skin—it also requires toning the tissues and muscles that underlie it, to prevent wrinkles and blemishes. Avoiding a large tummy, a "middle-age spread," is not only a question of losing fat, but also of strengthening the abdominal muscles, of straightening a tired vertebral column, and avoiding intestinal distension.

We can accomplish all this by using the simple method of applying pressure to specific points that correspond to certain areas of the body.

In using the pressure points for the purpose of promoting health and beauty, the technique will be a little different from that described in *How to Give Yourself Relief from Pain by the Simple Pressure of a Finger*. When we use finger pressure to bring relief from discomfort, we cease stimulation of the pressure point once the pain has disappeared. But in this book our aim is to *safeguard* and so to prevent, or to remove, chronic disorders, and we cannot expect instantaneous results.

Merely applying pressure from a fingertip will not make blackheads magically disappear, nor will it straighten a vertebral column before our very eyes. Patience is more important here than physical force. The points need to be stimulated without excessive effort, but regularly. The easiest way is to apply pressure two to three times a day—on first getting up in the morning and while getting ready for bed at night, for example—for two to three minutes at each session. It is useful to get into the habit of combining stimulation with the exercises and movements that we will describe in the course of this book. The effects will then be more rapid and the results even better.

So, if you have the will to go through the routine for a few minutes a day, you will have the pleasure over the weeks that follow of watching your blemishes disappear and your body become rejuvenated, and, even better, you will have learned how to prevent these disorders from appearing in the first place.

This, then, is the aim of this book. It will have been achieved once you have successfully *safeguarded* those two inseparable elements, your *health* and your *beauty*.

How to Use the Method

The method is very simple. First of all, you will need to locate the relevant pressure point. Once you have found it—with the aid of the photographs and drawings in this book—all you need to do is to place one of your fingers on the point and press down forcefully, vibrating or rotating your finger slightly. If you want to press even more precisely on the point, you could use a smaller object—the end of a pen or pencil, for example.

The method is almost the same as the one that I have described in *How to Give Yourself Relief from Pain by the Simple Pressure of a Finger* for easing discomfort. *However, there are two important differences that should be noted:*

To achieve relief from pain, you may need to apply pressure forcefully—but, if you are safeguarding your health, the pressure should be more gentle, especially when you are treating the face.

Pressure should cease once pain has disappeared—but, when the method is used to safeguard your health, it is important to realize that the results are not immediate.

You need to stimulate the relevant point for up to five minutes every day, and for certain conditions (for example, when treating cellulite) several times a day. Also, it is helpful to combine stimulation with certain muscular exercises and postural movements. Details of these are given in the pages that follow.

You may find it surprising that stimulation of some points can treat several conditions. This is simply because these points correspond to certain parts of the body, and stimulating them will help the various troubles that affect these different parts.

The Face

How to Preserve Your Youthful Looks, or How to Try to Recapture Them

Your face is your most important asset; it is your calling card. Your whole personality and individuality can be read in it. Your emotions and feelings are conveyed through your face, and you use it to communicate with the outside world.

And yet your face is more exposed than any other part of you to bad weather and climatic conditions. So there is nothing more important than caring for your face if it needs attention and taking all necessary steps to preserve this precious asset. It is quite unwise to think of facial problems as minor.

In the first part of this section, we shall look at the "real" diseases. In the second, we shall consider a number of unpleasant anomalies that affect the skin, its appearance and make-up. Also, however important the cutaneous covering, it is equally essential to care for the muscular foundation that forms and supports the shape of the face, as we have already pointed out. Surprisingly, works written by dermatalogical authorities do not usually consider the care of this muscular foundation. And yet, as the foundations grow weaker and sag, so the wrinkles and jowls appear. . . .

We shall now look at these different elements and discuss how to care for and preserve them by stimulating the relevant pressure points.

Acne

Acne can drive young people of both sexes to desperation, but it is not only an adolescent condition; sometimes it can last a lifetime. Acne spreads over the face in the form of a mass of purulent spots and causes considerable damage to the skin, and all this at an age when people are at their most self-conscious.

There are different varieties of acne; one sort manifests itself in a few scattered spots on the face and is not too great a problem. Another type covers the whole face with a rash of small suppurating heads. The worst is undoubtedly tuberculoid acne, which causes large boils; this can lead to considerable embarrassment for the sufferer in both professional and private life.

There are points that, if stimulated regularly, bring about a substantial improvement in acne. We will mention these points again, as they have a number of uses. One of them is on the hand, another on the wrist and the third on the ankle. Regular stimulation of each of these points for a few minutes two or three times a day should bring about a gradual improvement. One may also use the treatment recommended for associated conditions, which are described later.

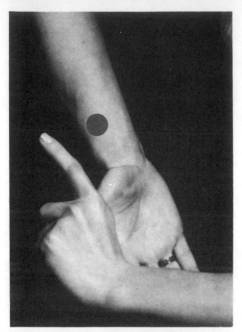

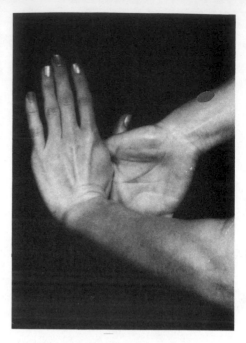

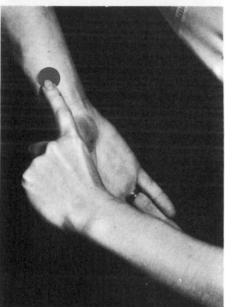

The point on the wrist is a very
important one for treating the head.
You can find it in the groove along
the fore-edge of the radius by locking
one thumb over the other thumb—
you will find that your index finger
held straight will indicate the
point exactly.

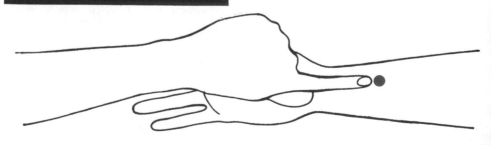

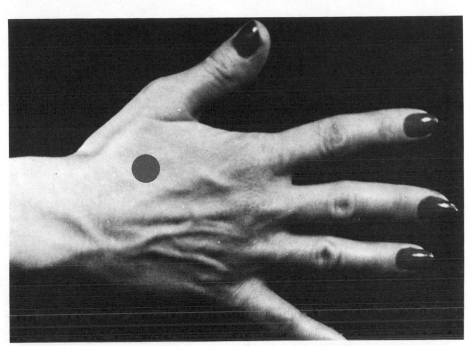

The second point is on the back of the
hand in the interstice between the
thumb and the index finger, exactly in
the hollow at the base of the bulge of
the metacarpal bone, which leads to
the finger.

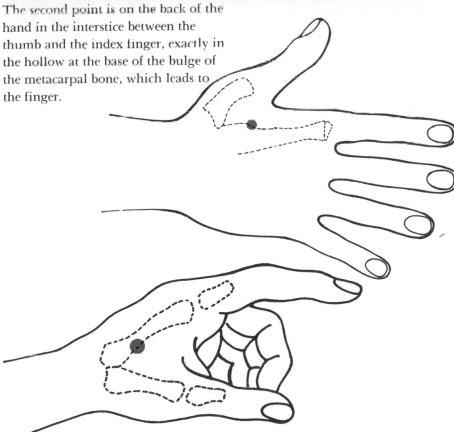

The third point is on the outside of
the ankle, one finger's width higher
than the protrusion above the joint.

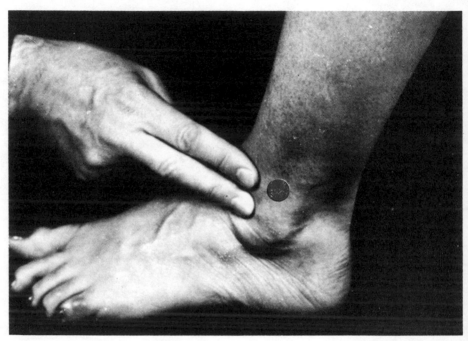

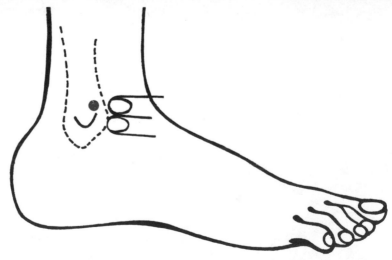

Blackheads

Blackheads are dried up secretions that block the outlets of the sebaceous glands. They appear as tiny blackish spots and, when pressure is applied around them, a tiny thread of whitish or yellowish substance can be squeezed out. They are particles of grease that have accumulated because the duct is blocked. If the accumulation is large, a small swelling called a comedo results.

This condition is usually associated with an excess of oily secretion, or sebum—which may have a number of causes. The main one is the way the hormones act on the glands during puberty and adolescence. The sebum may easily become infected, and infected blackheads can lead to acne. So acne usually begins with the appearance of blackheads.

In susceptible people blackheads may continue to appear during their entire lifetime, and the pressure of the retained secretions causes dilation of the skin pores. The end result may be a rough, coarse complexion, dotted with small lumps and craters, which is very unattractive to look at.

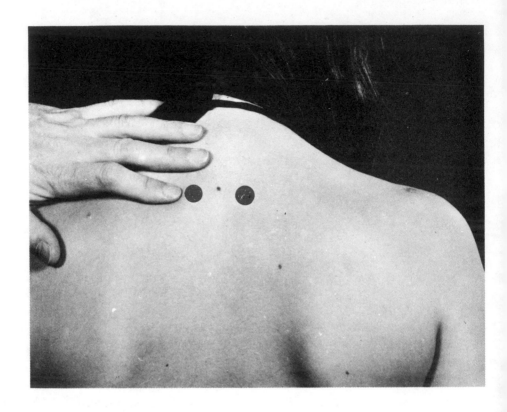

There is a point that can be
stimulated in an attempt to eliminate
blackheads. It is on the upper part of
the back, on either side of the vertebral
column, and is easy to find. First
locate the large swelling at the base of
the neck, which is the last cervical
vertebra, then move down, counting
the first three protrusions of the dorsal
vertebrae. The point is two fingers'
width away from the third protrusion,
on either side of the vertebral column.
It should be stimulated regularly, on
both sides, every morning and
evening, for two to three minutes.

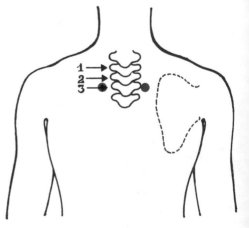

Acne Rosacea

This is a condition in which the face is streaked with tiny veins that run across the cheeks and nose. These little veins may remain unobtrusive, but they can look very ugly indeed if there are a number of them. Acne rosacea is a physical disability. It is often wrongly attributed to drunkenness, yet the poor sufferers are often teetotallers!

Two pressure points on the forearm are of great help in treating this. These points should be stimulated twice a day for two to three minutes.

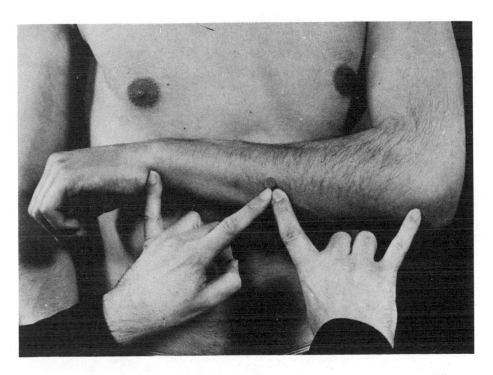

The first is on the back of the forearm, halfway along the bone called the ulna, which runs from the little finger to the elbow. Find the small nick in the bone and stimulate forcefully.

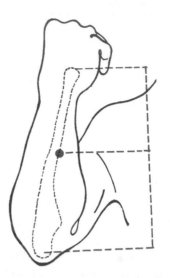

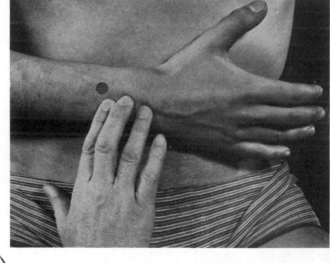

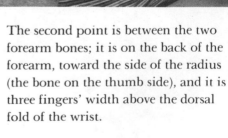

The second point is between the two forearm bones; it is on the back of the forearm, toward the side of the radius (the bone on the thumb side), and it is three fingers' width above the dorsal fold of the wrist.

Brown, Black, and White Blemishes

Spots on the face can cause embarrassment. They may be brownish, black, or white. Brown spots are sometimes called beauty spots or moles. In general they are not a problem but, if they are too numerous, they can look unpleasant, especially on a very pale skin.

Another variety are the spots which come with age. They are coffee-colored, brownish-blackish areas in the shape of irregular stains or blots. You should watch these carefully since they may develop into skin cancers.

Sometimes brown pigmentation can spread extensively—this may happen during pregnancy, for example, but it usually goes away after birth. (The pill can also cause this condition—chloasma, as it is known scientifically—and pigmentation caused in this way is indelible.) Such spots should be treated as soon as they appear.

The opposite of pigmentation—depigmentation—may occur. This happens when a generalized condition called *vitiligo*, about which little is known, affects the face. We will come across *vitiligo* again in a later chapter under the section that deals with general skin disorders.

One point is used to treat all such facial troubles, whether brown or black spots or depigmentation.

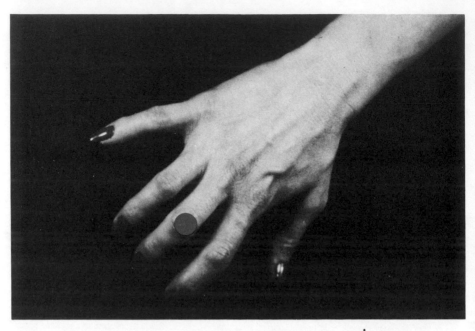

This point can be found on the back of the middle finger. When you bend this finger, the point is exactly in the center of the first joint. This point should be stimulated vigorously on both hands every day. After a short time, the various skin disorders should improve.

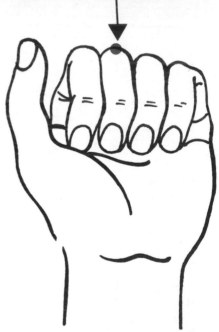

Another unpleasant problem occurs when women's faces become affected by excess hair. We will look at this in a later chapter, along with general excess hair problems.

Pale or Grayish Complexion

A face that is too pale and washed-out looking may be considered unattractive by some people. It sometimes happens people convalescing from an infectious illness have a literally gray complexion. This can also happen to people who have absorbed mercury or silver salts, which are present in certain medicines, or to those who are in occupations where they are exposed to these compounds.

But a pale complexion may simply be a result of physical constitution. In this case, the stimulation of specific pressure points can be very effective. There are three points. All of them should be stimulated two or three times a day for a few months.

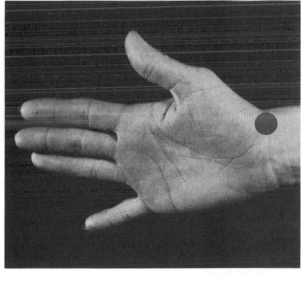

The first is on the edge of the fold of the wrist at the near end of the bone at the base of the thumb, where it joins the radius. This is sometimes known as the "anatomical snuff box" because snuff-takers in the past used to measure out their pinch of snuff into this hollow before sniffing it up.

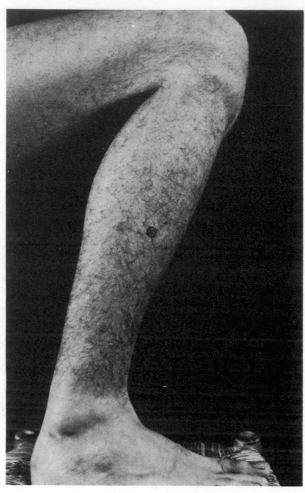

The second is on the outer side of the
leg muscle, four fingers' width above
the middle of a line joining the bend
of the knee to the outer edge of the
ankle.

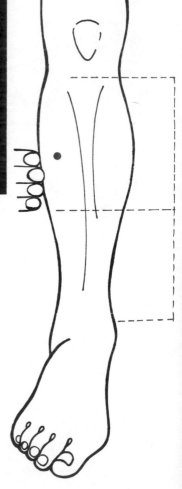

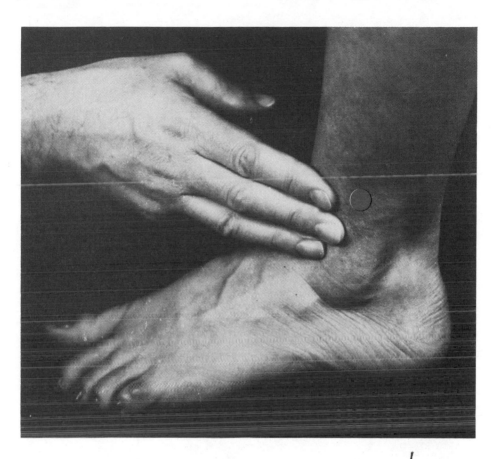

The third point is also on the outer edge of the leg, three fingers' width above the ankle. Stimulate it deeply and regularly.

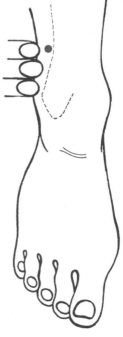

Rashes and Red Flushes

Now we shall look at red flushes. Our skin may become red temporarily after a large meal, for example, and some people are affected even after a light meal.

One point will bring fast relief.

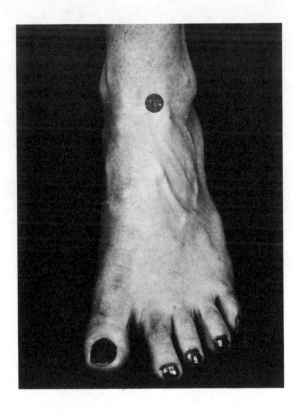

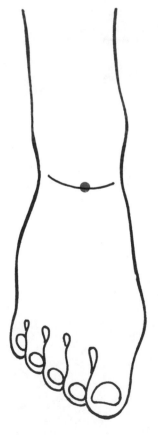

This point may be stimulated discreetly. It is in the middle of the dorsal fold of the foot. Massage it energetically for a few minutes.

Redness can also be an emotional reaction, caused by shyness or stage fright or a disagreeable situation.

Two points bring quick relief and can be stimulated equally discreetly.

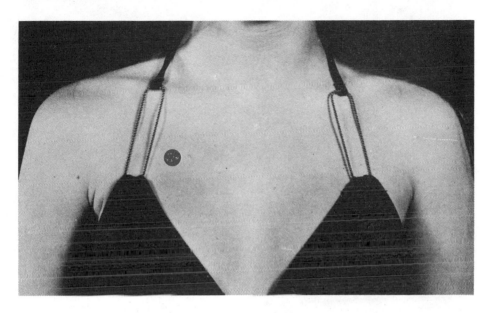

The first point is on the chest in the second intercostal space on the right-hand side, three fingers' width below the middle of the collar bone. Stimulate forcefully and the redness should disappear in a short time.

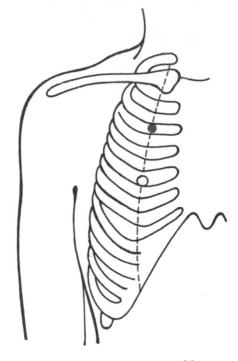

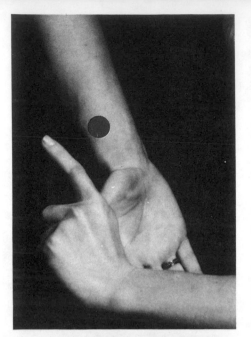

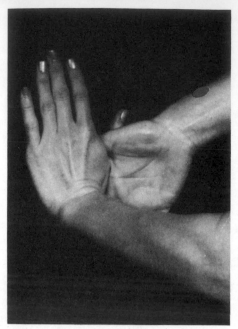

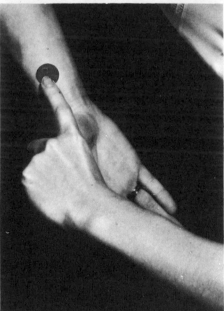

The second point is on the edge of the fold of the wrist at the near end of the bone at the base of the thumb. Regular stimulation on both wrists for two to three minutes will bring about a rapid improvement.

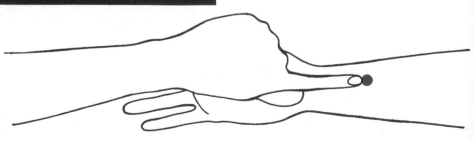

Oily or Dry Skin

The surface of the skin may be troublesome both esthetically (it is never pleasant to have a shiny face), and medically. An oily skin will easily become infected; acne or eczema may flourish, leaving obtrusive scars.

One might think that a dry skin would be better, but this is not necessarily so. A dry skin also produces secretions, often quite abundantly; but these secretions are too fluid, and evaporate too quickly, without time to moisturize and protect the skin.

Specific points, when stimulated, can act on the quality of secretion. There are two points for oily skin and one point for dry skin.

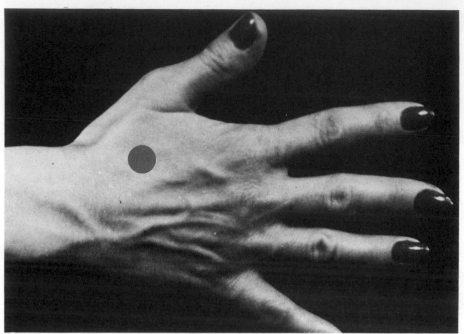

The first of these, for oily skins, is on the back of the hand in the space between the thumb and the index finger against the bone that leads to the index finger (the second metacarpal). Stimulate the point regularly.

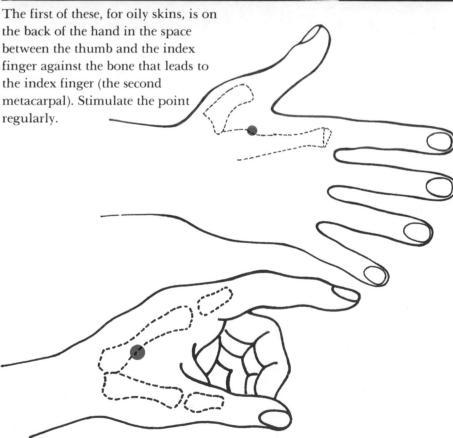

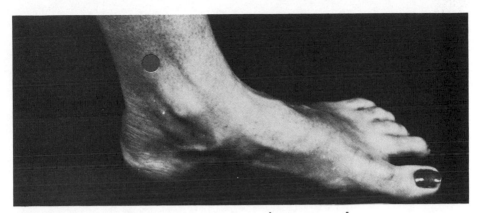

The second point for oily skins is on the inner side of the leg, three fingers' width above the ankle. Stimulate this point conscientiously for a few minutes every day. Gradually, you will observe an improvement in your skin.

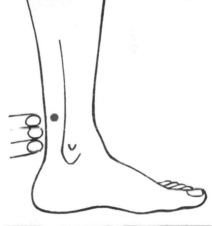

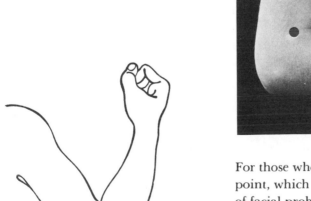

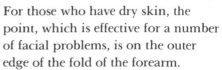

For those who have dry skin, the point, which is effective for a number of facial problems, is on the outer edge of the fold of the forearm.

How to Prevent and Treat Wrinkles

For those who want to safeguard their health and thereby their beauty, maintaining one's face and avoiding the ageing effects of wrinkles is a constant preoccupation.

As we have already pointed out, the youthfulness of the face does not depend merely on the state of the skin; the underlying facial muscles are of prime importance.

There are no fewer than seventeen principal facial muscles. These are known as the muscles of expression, and we use them, consciously or unconsciously, to express our ideas and feelings nonverbally.

We should look after these muscles regularly—at least once a day, as a normal part of our toilet—in much the same way as women put on make-up and men apply after-shave lotion.

When we care for these muscles, we are preserving the charm and freshness of our looks and avoiding the appearance of wrinkles and sagging skin. If these have already appeared, this treatment is an easy method of containing them, and sometimes even of making them go away; so it is *both a cure and a prevention*.

It is a striking fact that wrinkles on the face always appear in exactly the same places. They even have a name depending on their position and the type of expression they lead to (see diagram).

Consequently, we are able to use the same therapy for everyone who wants to prevent wrinkles or to remove them once they have started to appear.

We shall now consider this therapy in detail.

Among the Chinese—and few people have smoother faces—treatment of the face always involves the combination of stimulating a pressure point (one or several) and making a movement. These two are inseparable if treatment is to succeed.

We shall look at each part of the face from top to bottom, beginning with the forehead, the eyebrows, the nose, and then the cheeks (and their fallen companions, the jowls), and finally we shall end with the most important part of the face: the eyes and the surrounding area.

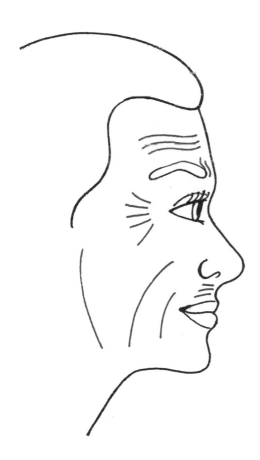

Wrinkles on the Forehead

The forehead is very mobile and flexible. Beauticians and sculptors are well aware of this. The forehead often develops a number of horizontal wrinkles running parallel to each other from the top of the eyebrows to the hair line. They are sometimes known as thought wrinkles—a little ironically perhaps. When you think something out deeply, you often frown, and this movement of the forehead muscles causes your brow to break into ridges.

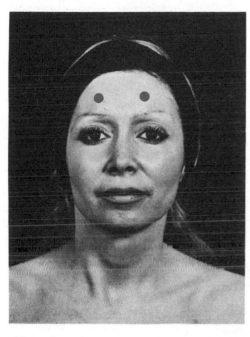

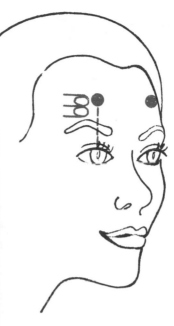

There is an important point that can prevent these wrinkles and may also cure them. This point is on the forehead, on either side of the median line, two fingers' width above the middle of the eyebrow.

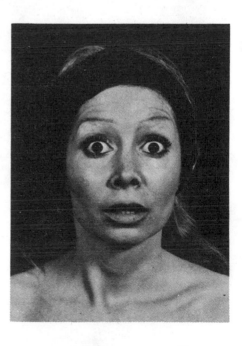

In front of your mirror, raise your eyebrows several times while stimulating the points. This exercise of simultaneously moving your forehead and stimulating the points is best done in the morning and evening for two to three minutes each time.

Maintain and Tone Your Eyebrows

The eyebrows define the area between the eyes, the forehead, and the top of the nose. This area is marked by two or three deep folds— important wrinkles that show when we are angry. If we are about to have an outburst of temper or to reprimand someone, we often frown, and these wrinkles become more marked. Sometimes they are known as adventurers' wrinkles, since it seems that they are particularly prominent among travelers. There are two points that are particularly effective in treating this area. Stimulate them deeply, while you systematically frown and then relax your eyebrows.

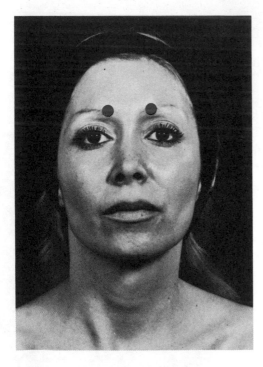

The first is at the inner end of the eyebrow in the small painful niche that you can feel with your finger.

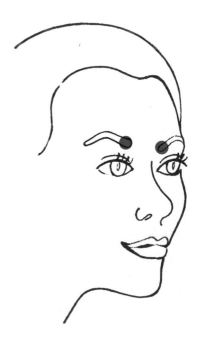

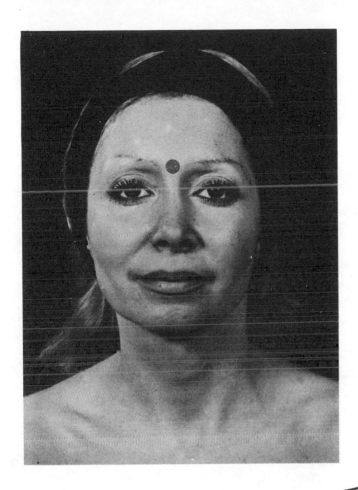

The second is on the bulge between the eyebrows known anatomically as the "glabella."

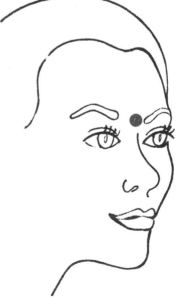

43

As we have said before, massage the
points and practice the movements we
have described for two to three
minutes morning and evening.

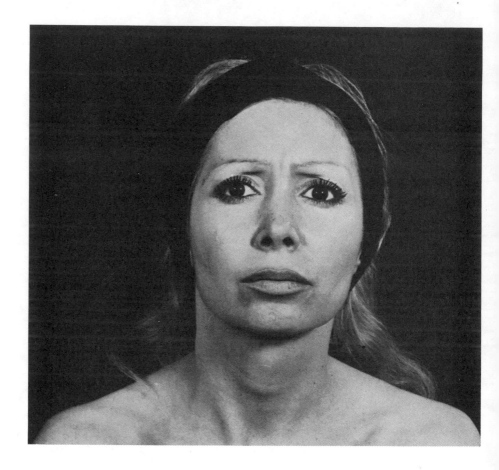

This is an excellent method of toning up the area and removing those
unattractive wrinkles that give a hard look to the face, especially as
they are often asymmetrical.

Wrinkles on the Nose

The nose by itself does not have any wrinkles, but on each side of the nose there is a long line, sometimes descending to the chin, which we have already shown in our general diagram. These have been called the martial wrinkles because they seem to be more common among soldiers and people who order others about.

There is a muscular exercise for the nose that can prevent and lessen the chance of these wrinkles appearing.

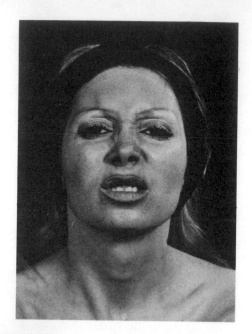

Try to contract the nose by lifting it with the muscles of your nostrils, moving them upward and outward, and accompany this movement with stimulation of two points.

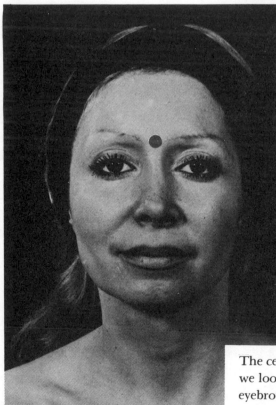

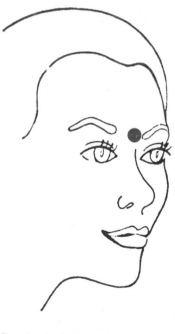

The central point is the same one that we looked at in the section on eyebrows; it is the point just under the "glabella," below the small swell of the frontal bone at the top of the nose.

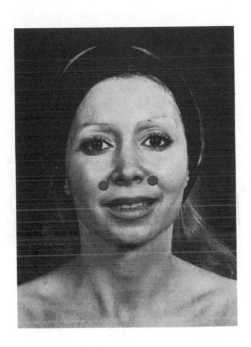

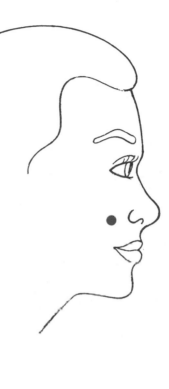

The other point is half a finger's
width outside the nostril.

The nostrils themselves can be physically unattractive. They may be too flared, or too narrow, giving the face a startled look in the former case, and a severe, or even evil, appearance in the latter. One simple movement will treat either of these deformities.

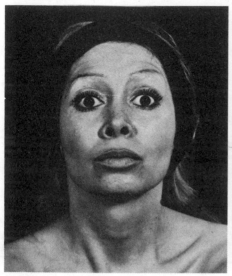 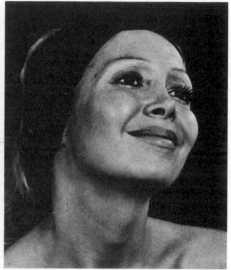

The movement involves the successive dilation and constriction of the nostrils—the wings of the nose.

Combine this with stimulation of the point at the end of the nostril, where it joins on to the rest of the face, on both sides.

Stimulate these two points for two or three minutes each morning and evening.

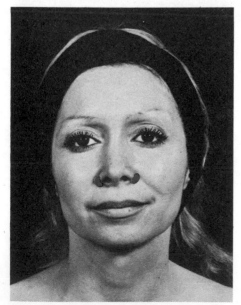 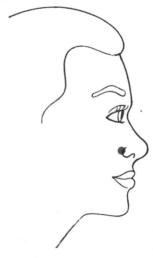

Maintaining and Toning the Cheeks and Preventing Jowls

We shall now consider the care of our cheeks. Cheeks determine the expression and the quality of the face. Young people have soft, delicate, supple cheeks; but, as we grow older, small wrinkles appear.

The important points can help safeguard the freshness of the cheeks; these points are essential to avoid sagging cheeks or jowls. Jowls are particularly unattractive.

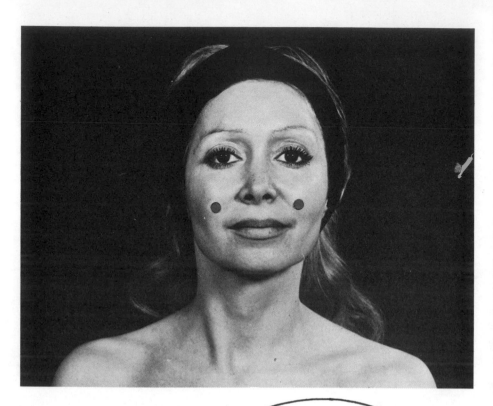

The first point is in a small niche immediately below the cheek line. Pressure on this point will be slightly painful because there is a sensitive nerve close by. Stimulate it for two or three minutes every morning and evening.

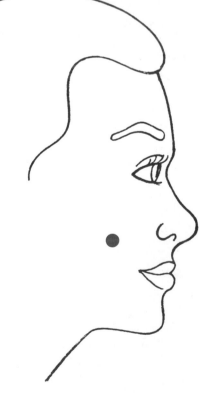

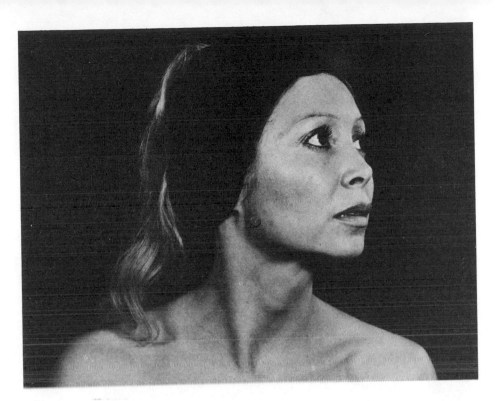

The second point is just underneath the jaw line. Again, the point will feel a little sensitive. Stimulate both points while alternatively puffing out and hollowing the cheeks: this will tone the cheek muscles and strengthen them. Stimulate for two or three minutes every morning and evening.

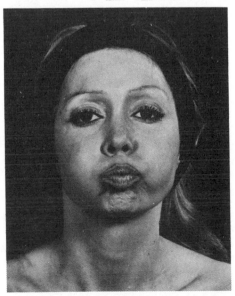

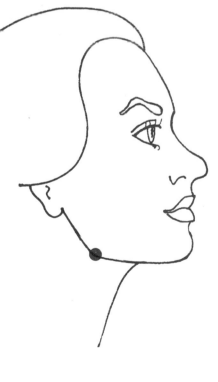

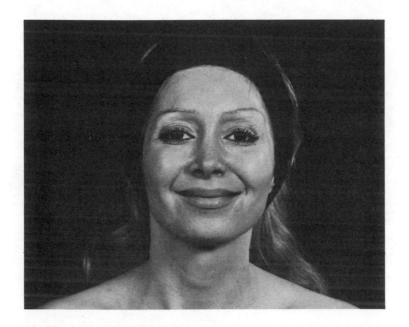

This exercise may be alternated with
another very simple one—smiling.
Smiling lifts the cheek muscles and
preserves their tone. For the most
effective use of this movement, smile,
keeping your mouth closed, every
morning and evening.

Wrinkles Around the Mouth and Lips

We shall first consider the mouth as a whole, then the lower and upper lips separately.

Let us look at the movements and points that are relevant to the area of the mouth.

These are two movements that can with benefit be repeated often.

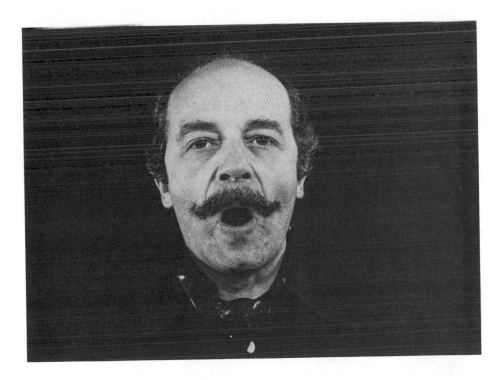

The first movement is shaping the mouth into a square by opening the lips wide apart.

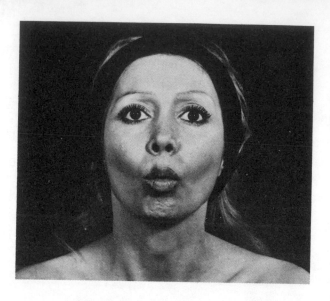

The second movement is a pouting outward of the lips—purse them forward as far as you can.

These two movements are associated with two points. These two points should be stimulated with two fingers every morning. This will bring great benefit to the skin around the mouth.

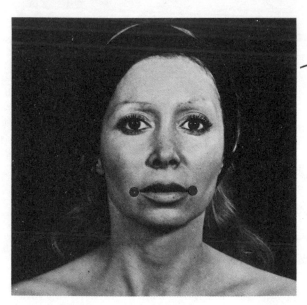

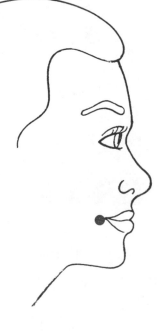

The first point is half a finger's width outside the corner of the lips on each side of the face.

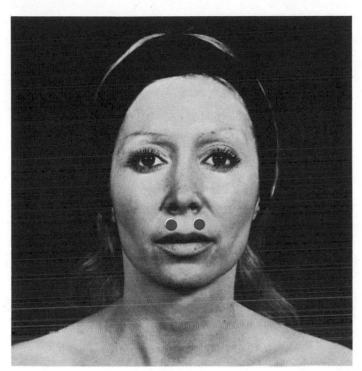

The second point is above the upper
lip, halfway between the bottom of
the nose and the upper edge of the lip.

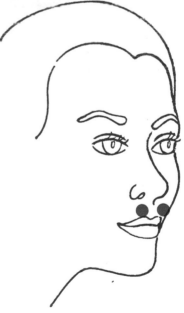

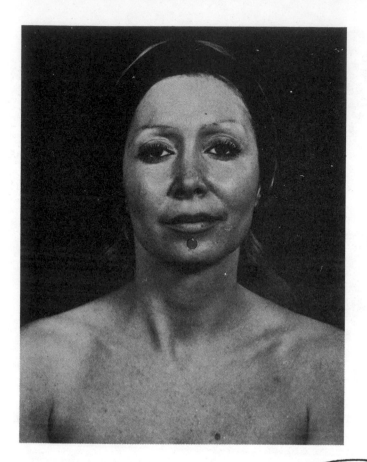

When treating the lower lip you should use retraction and protrusion movements—rather as we do when speaking. At the same time, stimulate the point that is immediately below the lower lip in the sub-labial dimple.

Repeat at least twice a day, and more often if possible.

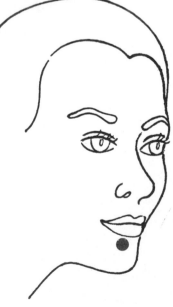

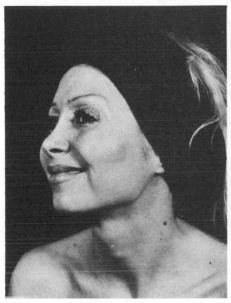
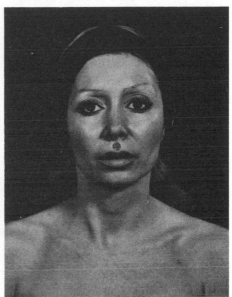

A wrinkle may form on the upper lip, sometimes known as the "toothless wrinkle" because it usually occurs in those who no longer have teeth, or who have a poorly fitting denture.

To treat this, retract and then protrude the lips while stimulating a point in the middle of the fold of skin halfway between the top of the lips and the nose.

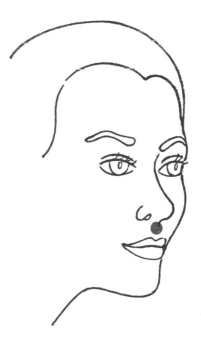

Wrinkles and Bags Around the Eye

Your eyes give expression to your face depending on your mood. They widen with joy, with wonder or anger; they shine or look dull according to your mental state.

There are movements and points that are particularly effective for the eyes.

We shall look first at the general treatment, and then at the treatment of the peripheral area—that is, the upper lid, the lower lid, and the outer corner.

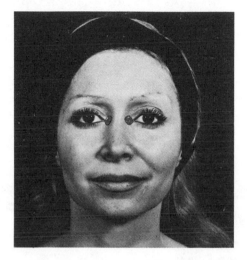

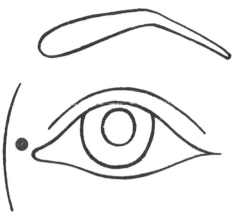

The principal point that will help an infected eye, as well as protect a healthy one, is in the inner corner of the eye above the small swelling known as the lachrymal caruncle, from which our tears flow.

Stimulate this point deeply while gazing far into the distance at an imaginary horizon. You will be improving the general tonicity of the eye, as well as its brightness. The point acts on the conjuctiva and the cornea, and is thus able to modify the luster of the eye itself.

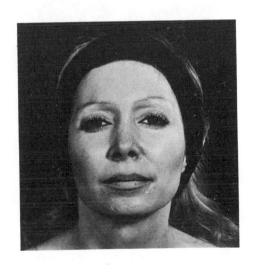

Let us now consider the upper and lower lids separately. There are two points which are effective for the upper lid and which prevent wrinkling and flabbiness.

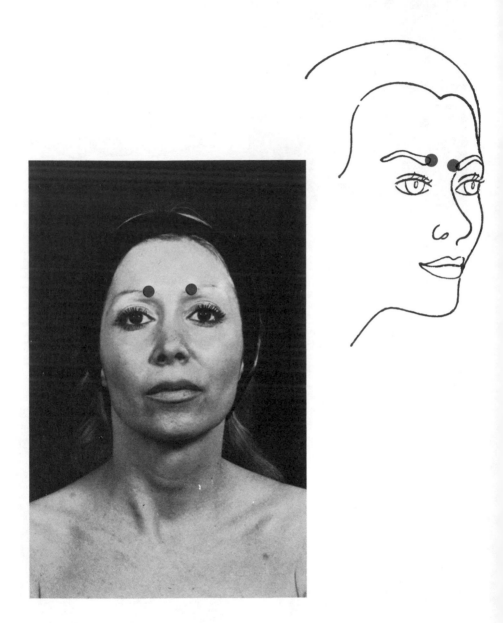

We have already come across the first point. It is on the inner end of the eyebrow in the sensitive niche.

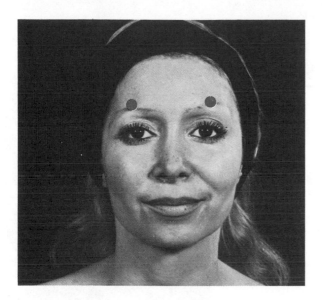

The second point is in the middle of the eyebrows, in the midst of the hairs.

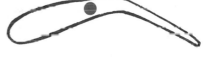

Stimulate these two points deeply for two to three minutes while blinking the lid. This action should prevent flabbiness of the surrounding skin area.

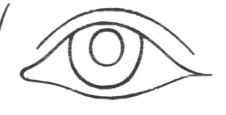

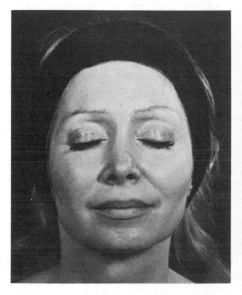

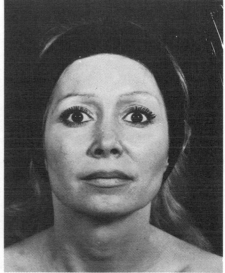

Let us now look at the two points for the lower lid.

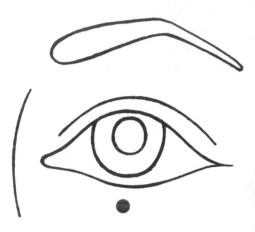

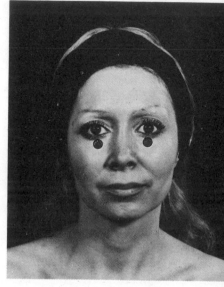

The first point is in the middle of the lower edge of the eye socket—once again in a small hollow just below the pupil when the subject is gazing ahead.

Stimulate regularly for two or three minutes.

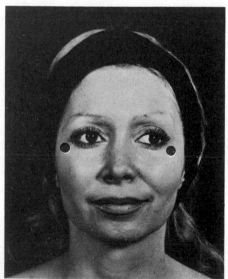

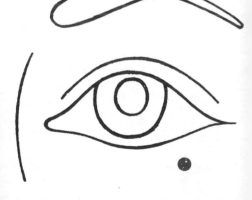

The second point is one finger's width outside the first. These two points combat heavy eyelids and the bags underneath them that are so unsightly. They also treat the wrinkles under the eye, which may be numerous, and they improve rings under the eyes that often occur due to lack of sleep.

The outer edge of the eye should also be looked after with care. This is the area where several tiny wrinkles, sometimes known as "crow's feet," may appear—they may be particularly ugly as they can age even a relatively youthful looking face.

Two points are important. Stimulate them while blinking your lids, as before. Thus "crow's feet" wrinkles can be prevented or reduced in number if they have already appeared.

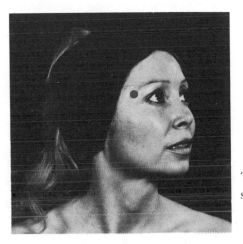

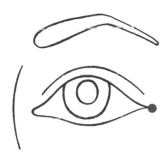

The first is on the outer side of the eye socket.

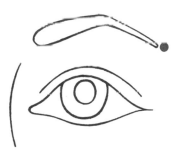

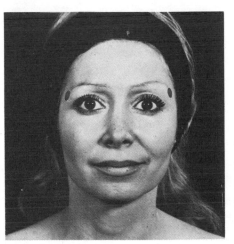

The second is just beyond the tail of the eyebrow, in a tiny depression in the bone, which can easily be felt with a finger.

All these movements and stimulation should be practiced every morning and evening. But it is a good idea to practice them for a few minutes during the day as well.

Hair Care

Introduction

Your hair is your crowning feature, the natural frame for your face. This is the reason why, from earliest times, people have paid the utmost attention to hair care.

What exactly is hair? Hair grows from a deep root in the dermis and its matrix; the particular point right at the base of the root is known as the papilla. As it grows from the papilla, the hair swells into a bulb shape—this is the whitish swelling that you can see when you pull a hair out of your scalp. The bulb continues into a sort of receptacle or follicle. Then the hair pushes through the epidermis, and this section, which pierces the skin, is known as the stem or shaft. Once it has pushed through the scalp it follows its natural inclination.

A small muscle, which can make the hair stand on end, is attached to each hair follicle. Opening into every hair follicle are sebaceous glands, which secrete an oily substance called sebum. Sebum is the lubricant that allows the hair to slide freely through the skin of the scalp and also waterproofs and protects it. Sebum may also be the cause of trouble—if there is too little sebum the hair is dry and brittle; if there is too much the hair becomes oily.

The state of our hair reflects the condition of the body. Beautiful hair implies general good health.

There are about 100,000 hairs on the human head. In general, they have a life of four to five years. Then they grow again. The growing phase is long, and lasts about four years; it is known scientifically as the anagene phase. It is followed by the telogene, or rest, phase of the hair, which lasts approximately six months. Finally, the hair falls out, the root rises, and a new hair takes its place—at least in the normal way of things.

Of course, hair varies from one individual to another—in quantity, in appearance (straight, curly, or frizzy) and in thickness (thick, wiry, or fine). All these differences should be taken into account.

The two major troubles that affect the hair are hair loss and graying with age.

We shall now consider these problems.

How to Prevent or Slow Down Loss of Hair

Hair can fall out either in patches, or all over. There are a number of causes of baldness: traumatism, burns, shock, exposure to X rays, treatment by certain drugs, infectious diseases (especially fevers), or parasites. Scalp diseases such as ringworm may be common in schools.

Alopecia

Hair loss in round or oval patches is known as alopecia. At its worst, the entire scalp becomes bald. It seems that alopecia has a purely nervous, psychological cause, and it can come on suddenly. It sometimes occurs hours or minutes after a piece of bad news, a shock, or a feeling of anxiety. Dermatologists often treat alopecia with tranquilizers and injections of strong steroid drugs but, if you want to avoid this, there are particular pressure points for treating alopecia—these are known as the anguish points. They should be stimulated for several minutes two or three times every day.

They are:

First, points on the inside bend of the wrist.

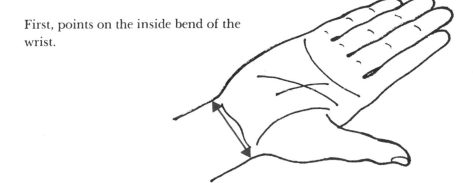

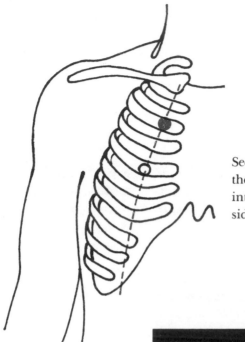

Second, the general anguish point, on the mammary line in the second intercostal space on the right-hand side.

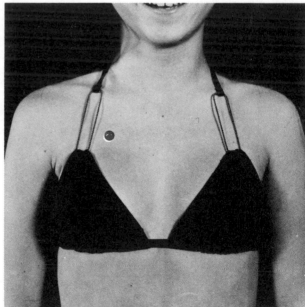

Baldness

Total loss of hair is common. This may be merely temporary; some or all of the hair may be lost after an illness, treatment with certain drugs, a period of fatigue, or after pregnancy, for example. However, the most common form of baldness is male pattern baldness. But women, particularly those who take the pill, can experience hair loss, which may, rarely, be irreversible.

Many of us first experience loss of some hair at quite an early age. Baldness starts in specific areas—at the temples, where the hair recedes gradually, and on the crown of the head, the "tonsure." These three bald spots gradually increase in size until they meet each other. A mere semi-circle of hair remains, at the sides and back. In modern transplants hair from the peripheral section where hair remains is replanted along the central part. It will usually take fairly well.

But, before resorting to this drastic method, there are more gentle means of treatment that can be tried. These methods are more likely to be effective if they are used regularly. Two points are helpful for treatment of hair loss. If you stimulate them regularly, you may be able to arrest male pattern baldness temporarily or even stop it developing completely.

The first is on the inside of the bend of the knee at the back of the leg in the middle of the crease.

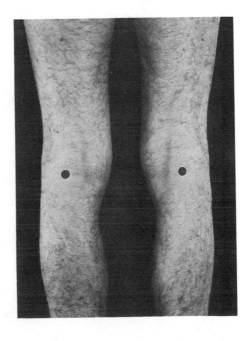

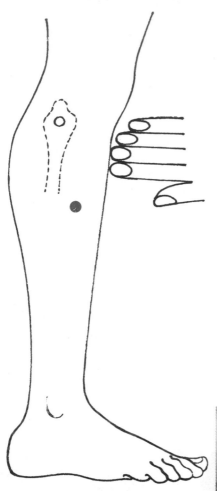

The second is on the outer side of the leg, a hand's width underneath the small swelling that is known as the head of the fibula—right in the middle of the outer muscle mass of the leg. (The fibula is the long thin bone on the outer side of the leg that starts at the knee in a small swelling.)

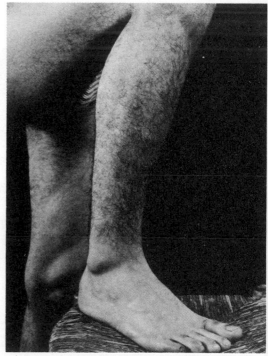

Gray or White Hair

Graying or whitening of the hair in humans, as in animals, is a sign of aging. It is caused by a chemical change in the structure of the hair, causing it to lose its pigment, and so its color. Hereditary factors are often significant; we all know of people who are completely gray by the age of thirty, and we also know old men who do not have a single gray hair.

External factors are also important; as with alopecia, an emotion or a physical or psychological shock can trigger off or accelerate graying of the hair. (We occasionally hear of people whose hair turns white overnight.)

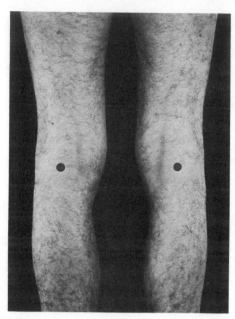

Graying can be restrained by using the same points that are described for the treatment of baldness; one is in the middle of the bend of the leg at the back of the knee.

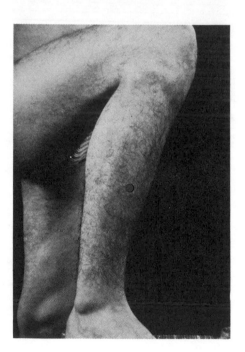

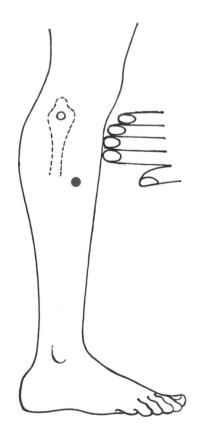

The other is on the outer side of the leg.

Oily or Dry Scalp

Apart from hair loss or alteration in hair color, the scalp itself may be ill, and any disorder here will affect the state of the hair. Seborrheic dandruff is very common and is caused by excessive secretion of sebum, the normal lubricant of the hair.

Sebum may be too abundant and too thick, in which case the scalp is too oily; it greases the fingers and the comb and loosens flakes of skin from the epidermis, forming dandruff. The sebum may also be inadequate and the scalp too dry; the normal lubrication is lost, and the hair is stiff, dull, and lifeless.

These unpleasant troubles can affect either sex from adolescence onward. Help can come from two pressure points. Massage them two or three times a day for a few minutes.

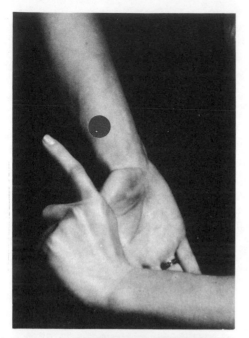

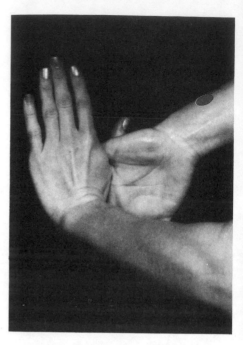

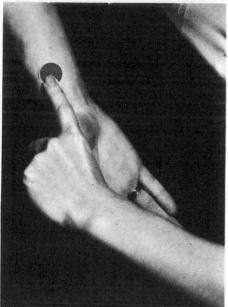

The first is on the wrist. You can find it in the groove along the fore edge of the radius by locking one thumb over the other thumb, and you will find that your index finger held straight will point exactly to the spot.

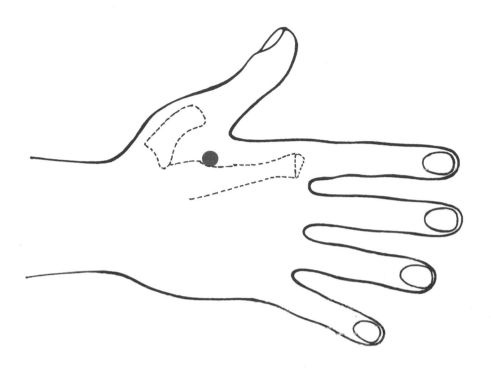

The second is on the back of the hand
at the angle of the second metacarpal,
the bone that leads to the index finger.

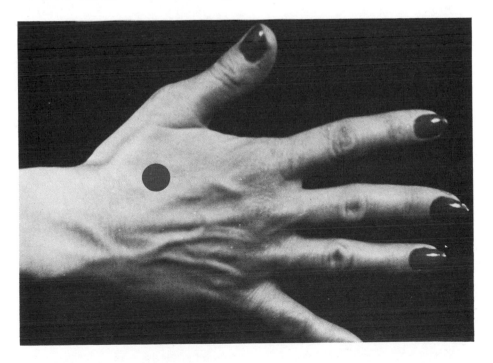

Neck, Shoulder, and Arms

How to Care for and Safeguard Your Neck

Esthetic defects of the neck are often linked to diseases that affect the organs in the neck, particularly the thyroid gland.

Any swelling in the neck requires medical advice. It may be an enlargement of the thyroid gland, a goiter, or an enlargement of the lymph glands, sometimes as a result of tonsillitus. In any event, consult your doctor. Goiters demand complex treatment—medical or surgical—which is outside the scope of this book.

The most common esthetic defect of the neck is sagging skin, which, as with the face, occurs with age, and creates unpleasant wrinkles. Deformities of the vertebral column, caused by age or arthritus, may also cause the skin of the neck to wrinkle. You will need to give attention to the nape of the neck to correct this. We shall see in a later chapter how to treat the vertebral column.

As for the wrinkles themselves, the combination of movements and stimulation of pressure points should improve the situation.

To tone the neck muscles, practice rotating the head first in one direction and then in the other. Roll the head as if were an enormously heavy sphere placed at the top of your body.

At the same time, you should also stimulate two points for two or three minutes two or three times a day.

The first point is at the back of the
elbow, at the part that is painful when
knocked; it is known as the funny
bone.

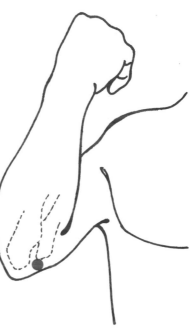

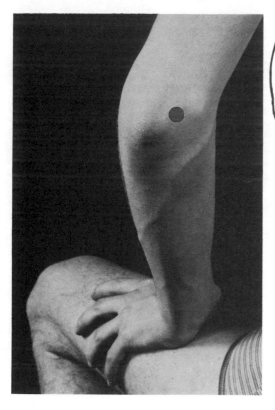

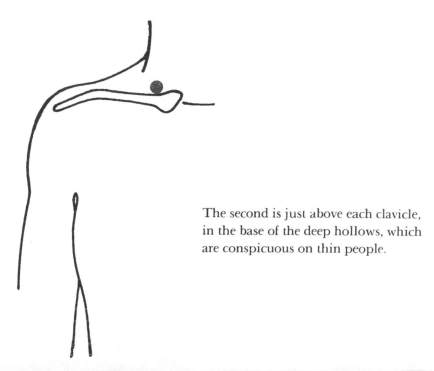

The second is just above each clavicle, in the base of the deep hollows, which are conspicuous on thin people.

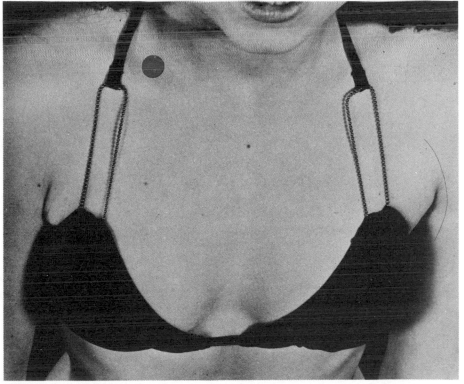

How to Safeguard the Shoulders and Arms

The tops of the upper arms are often obese on people of both sexes.

This localized obesity is caused by excess adipose tissue. It manifests itself in the form of a thickening of flesh at the top of the arm and the shoulder.

Both the arm and shoulder can be treated by four points.

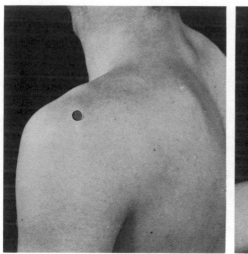 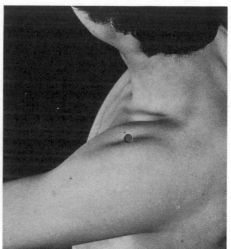

Two of them are on either side of the prominence above the head of the humerus, which is formed by the joint between the outer end of the clavicle (collar bone) and the scapula (shoulder blade).

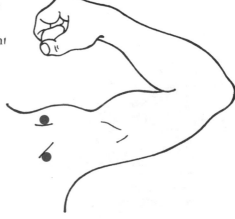

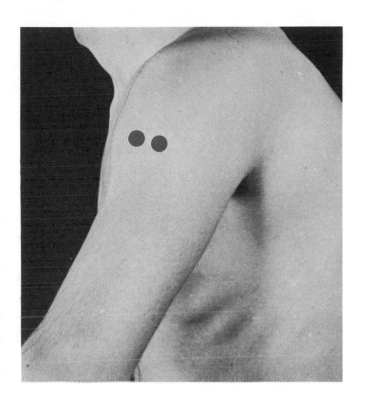

The two other points are either side of the intersection of the deltoid muscle—the muscle that covers and gives a round shape to the shoulder. Below it there is a sort of V-shaped groove; you should regularly stimulate the two extremities of the V. After some time, the arm and shoulders should gradually slim down. Of course, all the movements and exercises that build up the muscle in these two areas are useful. They can be combined with massage of the points we have just described.

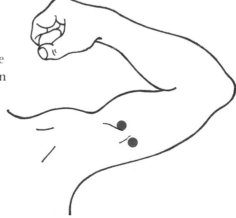

The Hand

How to Look After Your Hands

After the face, your hands—through their strength combined with their delicacy of gesture—best express your personality. But because of the many uses to which they are put and the dangers to which they are exposed, they are vulnerable to injury and to wear. We shall examine their treatment in the sections that follow, looking at the hand itself, the fingers, and the nails.

Our hands may be too thick or too big. These deformities are sometimes hereditary. But they may also be caused by diseases, some of which may be quite serious, such as those which originate from the pituitary gland—acromegaly, for example, in which the hands may enlarge greatly—or those that are of pulmonary origin when the ends of the fingers may swell, to resemble drumsticks. These diseases need medical care, and they are not our concern here.

However, if deformation of the hand is due to rheumatism, two points are effective. Stimulate them for a few minutes two or three times a day.

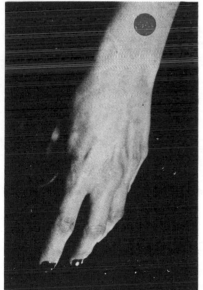

The first is on the back of the wrist, at the junction of the two bones of the forearm, two fingers' width above the skin crease at the back of the wrist joint.

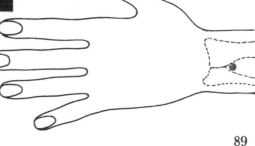

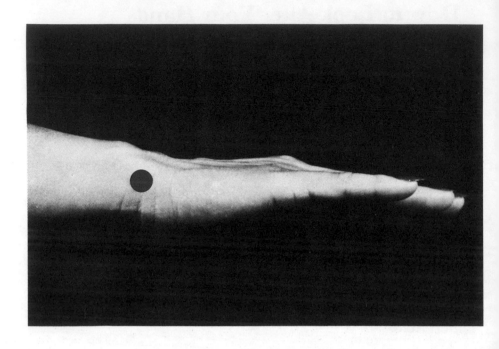

The second is on the inner edge of the wrist, close to the little finger, a little forward of the bend.

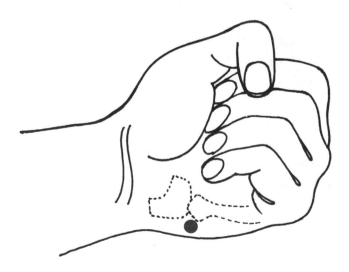

Deformed Fingers

Fingers may also be deformed. Deformation is almost always caused by rheumatism, whether it be degenerative rheumatism, arthritis due to age, or the more acute conditions of inflammatory rheumatism. Arthritis is the commonest cause of finger deformities. It begins with a painful swelling of the joints. Later, small, hard, bony lumps known as nodules appear, and at this stage the pain usually ceases but the deformity remains.

Relief may be obtained by pressure applied to different points.

These points are on the backs of the
fingers, at the middle of the first
knuckle joint.

Begin with the ring finger, then the
index, then the middle finger, then
the little finger, and finally the
thumb; always stimulate the points in
this order following the routine used
by the Chinese.

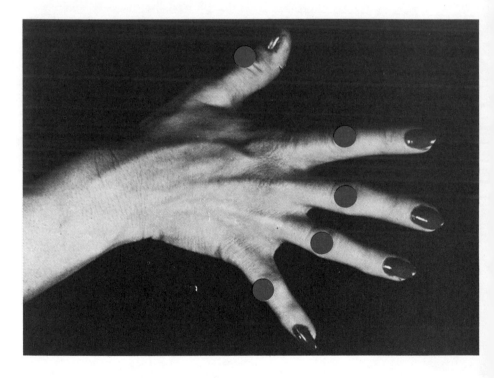

Each finger should be stimulated for a
few minutes two or three times a day.
If the fingers are very deformed by
rheumatism, stimulation should last
longer.

How to Make Your Nails Beautiful

Everyone should give constant care to nails. Everything external, in particular nail varnish, is merely cosmetic and can only hide the blemishes underneath. The nail, like hair, begins from a matrix beneath the skin, so we need an internal treatment. In the context of internal treatment, we shall study three particular elements.

1 The Shape of the Nail

When the nail becomes deformed and takes on a convex shape, this is usually symptomatic of a chronic pulmonary infection. If, on the other hand, the nail becomes concave, "spoon-shaped," this may be due to anemia, or it may be a hereditary trouble, in which case very little can be done to remedy it. Either sort of deformity indicates the need for medical attention.

The nail may also become deformed into ridges, either across the axis of the finger, or longitudinally, in the same direction as the finger. These deformities may be very upsetting, for men as much as for women, and can be treated with pressure points.

2 The Consistency and Strength of the Nail

The nail may become soft or very brittle, and the ends tend to split.

There are several reasons for this. It may be caused by a fungal infection, a variety of ringworm, or by the generalized skin disease psoriasis, in which case medical help should be sought.

3 The Color of the Nails

Whitish streaks running across or lengthways may appear on the nails. They may indicate serious illness or poisoning, whether external (e.g. arsenic) or internal (e.g. uremia, diabetes, etc.). But, more often, small white spots known scientifically as leuconychies appear; they have no serious significance. These are the whitish spots which we try to hide with nail polish.

Two points are very effective in treating the nails, with the exception of the serious or hereditary deformations, which we have already mentioned. Stimulating these points for a few minutes every morning and evening, one after the other, you should find that, although the existing white marks will not disappear, they will grow out with the nail, and recurrence will be prevented.

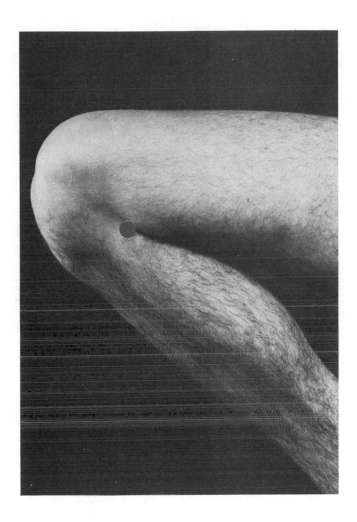

The first point is on the underside of
the bend of the knee, on the outer side
of the leg.

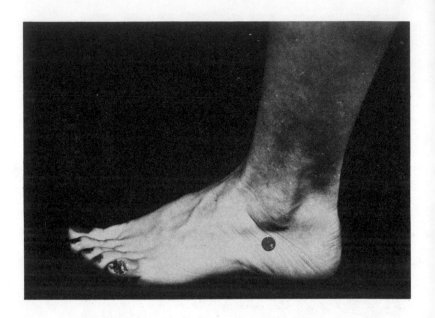

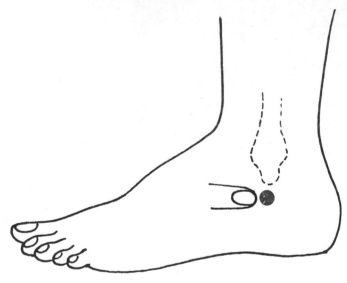

The second point is on the outer edge
of the ankle, half a finger's width
below the protrusion of the bone.

How to Stop Biting Your Nails

The unpleasant childhood habit of nail biting, which often drives parents to despair, can last into adult life.

This failing may become a social disability. The nails are deformed; the underlying skin, no longer protected by its natural covering, becomes irritated; sores, and even infections, develop.

There are two points that will bring relief to nailbiters.

The first point is on the underside of the bend of the knee, on the outer side of the leg.

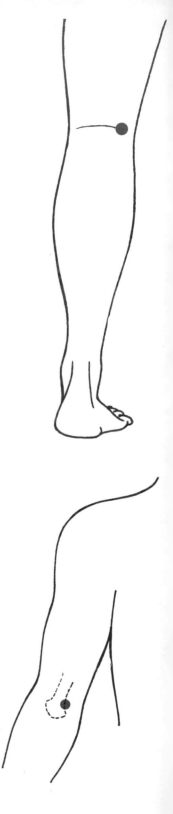

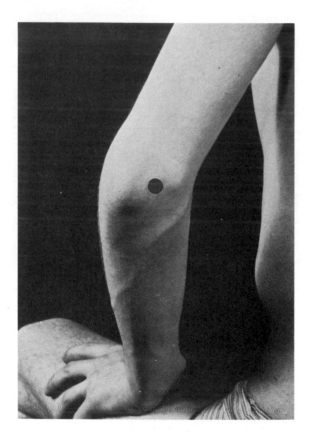

The other point is immediately behind the elbow joint, above the bony part called the olecranon, which forms the prominent sharp point of the elbow when it is bent.

Breasts

Safeguard the Health and Beauty of Your Breasts

Women's breasts, which are very important features of their bodies, may lose their shape and become deformed in different ways:

—deformations affecting the entire breast
—deformations affecting only the nipple and the surrounding area, the areola

The Entire Breast
There are two sorts of malformation: lack of size and excess size.

Breasts that are too small are usually like this as a result of glandular disturbances in the woman's body, possibly genetic in origin.

Breasts may also be too large as a result of glandular troubles, plus an excess of fatty tissues that makes them overprominent and heavy. For those who are so burdened, these excessively large breasts are a constant source of distress.

It is simply not possible to improve the shape through gymnastics, since the breast does not contain any muscle apart from some tiny fibers round the nipple. The only muscle is behind it, attached to the front of the ribs. The gland is directly beneath the skin, so, if it becomes too heavy, there is nothing to support it.

The Nipple

The breast terminates in a central, symmetrical, harmoniously raised part, the nipple. The shape of the nipple can be altered temporarily by nerve impulses or hormones, as when feeding a baby, but it can also be permanently retracted, as if swallowed up by the mass of the breast itself. This is called the umbilication or retraction of the nipple.

Two points are very effective for improving the shape of the breasts. They improve breasts that are too large or too small, as well as counteracting retraction of the nipple. Stimulate these points for a few minutes several times a day.

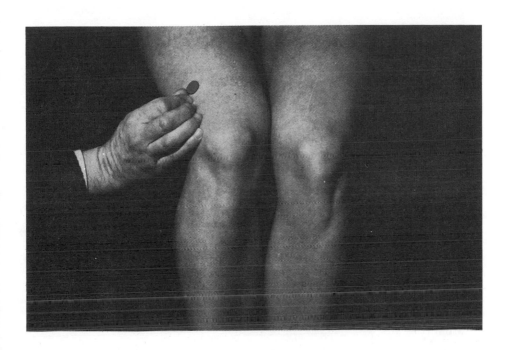

The first point is on the front side of
the thigh, five fingers' width above the
outer angle of the knee cap.

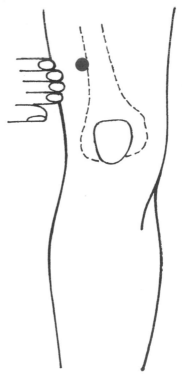

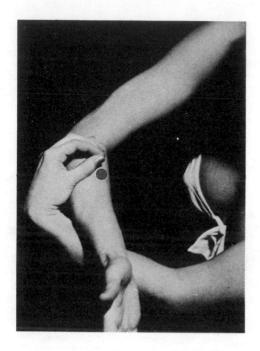

The second point is on the outer edge
of the forearm, three fingers' widths
below the bend of the elbow.

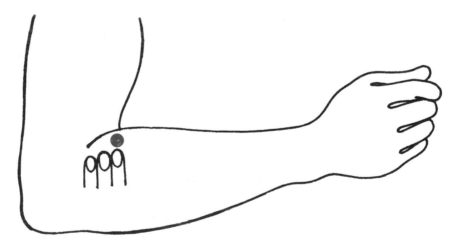

These two points are effective for all breast complaints, but we are, of
course, talking only about benign conditions, such as the painful
breasts that sometimes occur in young women before a menstrual
period. A doctor should always be consulted about the nature of any
breast complaint that lasts more than a day or two.

Cellulite

How to Avoid and Reduce Cellulite
on the Hips, Buttocks, Thighs, and Knee

Cellulite can be very unpleasant and particularly affects women.

What is cellulite?

Cellulite is a form of subcutaneous infiltration that deforms the figure and occurs nearly always in the female; it causes the flesh to swell irregularly with little lumps and hollows and sometimes small varicosities.

The following characteristic of the skin is an indication that it is affected by cellulite. When normal skin is pinched between thumb and fingers, it will appear pitted (so-called orange-peel skin): this does not indicate cellulite but is the appearance of perfectly normal, healthy skin. Cellulite, on the contrary, is made up of fatty packets underneath the skin in the above-mentioned areas—the hips, buttocks, and thighs.

Cellulite consists of packets of fat and is not just the result of water retention, as used to be thought. All the histological examinations of the body in these areas prove it.

This fat seems to be exactly the same chemically as the fat covering other parts of the body: what makes it different is its physiology. This fat will not melt, so to speak. The patient may diet and undergo severe slimming cures that will melt the fat everywhere else, and even reduce the size of the muscles, but the cellulite remains unaffected. Cellulite may even affect people who are otherwise very thin, producing an inappropriate exaggeration of certain parts of the figure. Cellulite then is fat, normal fat, but with a special physiology that excludes it from the normal metabolic processes. This physiology seems to be hereditary, possibly linked to the female chromosomes, since it is nearly always women who are affected.

The regular stimulation of specific points will help. The usual points relevant to obesity should also be used, but specific points that correspond to the affected areas of the body are equally important.

Among these points, we shall now look successively at those affecting:

—the buttocks
—the hips
—the thighs
—the knees

Cellulite on the Buttocks

Points that can decrease cellulite on the buttocks are on the sacrum, the bottom bone of the vertebral column, and are in two rows.

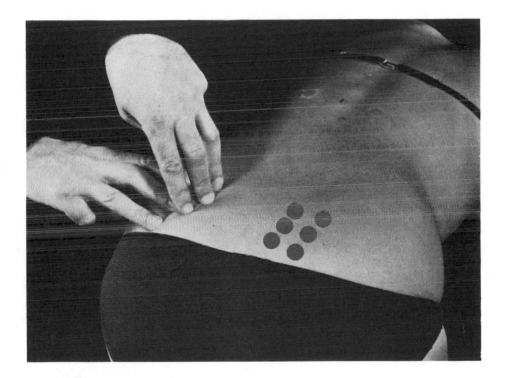

The first row of points is two fingers' widths from the median line that runs upward from the anus, between the buttocks. As the photo shows, stimulation should be performed with three fingers of the hand. The fingers stimulate each of the points. Repeat this exercise several times a day.

The second row of points is four fingers' width from the same median line. Again, using three fingers, stimulate in the same way. Repeat several times a day.

Cellulite on the Hips

The point is on the buttock, behind the hip joint. This is the same point as that which is effective for painful hips.

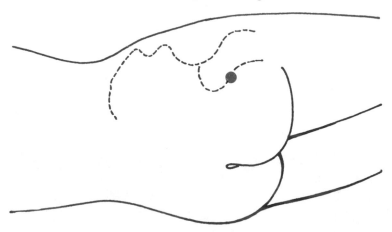

To locate the point on each side of the body, place the thumb on the highest part of the bony prominence, the iliac crest. Placing the rest of the hand on the thigh with the fingers slightly apart, the little finger will indicate the point, which should be stimulated several times a day.

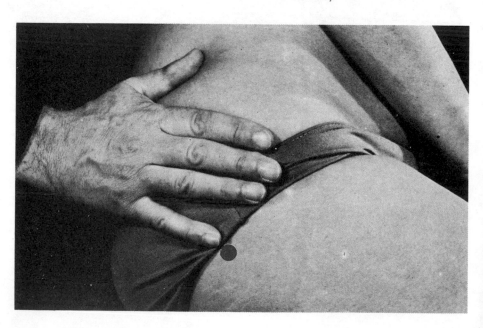

Cellulite on the Thigh

The points are on the front and back of the thigh. Stimulate them with the fingers of both hands.

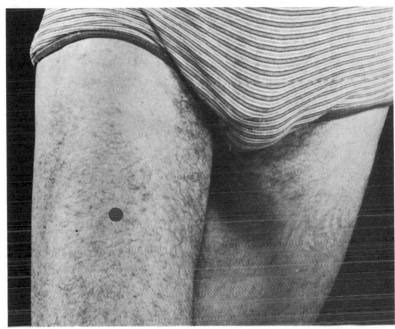

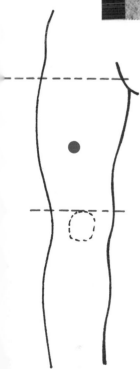

The one on the front is a hand's width below the iliac crest (the highest part of the pelvic basin). Place the heel of the hand against the iliac crest and point downward with the rest of the hand. You will find the point a little above the middle of the thigh.

The point behind is in the middle of the thigh.

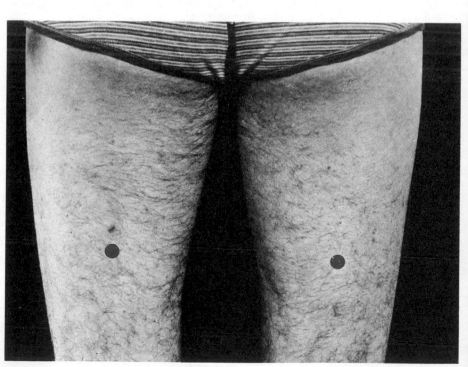

Cellulite on the Knee

There are two points that are effective for the knee.

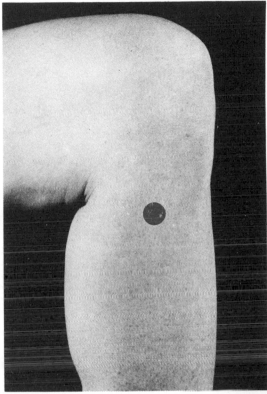

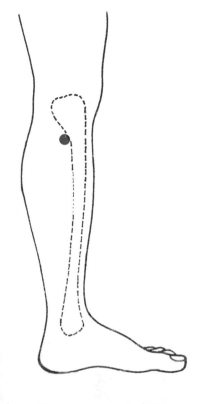

The first is just below the knee joint in the angle between the head and body of the tibia.

The second is above the external angle of the knee cap, three fingers' width from a vertical line that passes through the side of this bone.

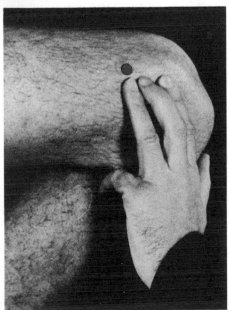

The Legs and Feet

Safeguard Your Legs, and Avoid Varicose Veins and Swelling of the Ankles

We shall now consider the leg and the complaints that may affect it. We have already treated the problem of cellulite. Cellulite does not affect the lower leg. Swellings that may occur are caused by other factors.

There is no cellulite from the lower knee region downward. Complaints of the legs are directly linked to the blood vessels that run through them. The entire esthetic of the leg depends on good circulation. In the legs, as indeed throughout the body, there are three sorts of circulation: arterial, venous, and lymphatic. Each of these has a different function. The arteries bring oxygenated blood to the extremities of the limb, the veins carry back the partly de-oxygenated, used blood to the heart, while the lymph vessels pump the fluids in the interstitial spaces between the cells back to the main vessels. We know that each of these three circulatory systems combines with and complements the other, and they interpenetrate to create a circulatory unity in the lower leg. Yet diseases of each part of this system are different. Affections of the arteries produce different complaints from conditions affecting the veins, for example. We shall now look at the different circulatory troubles that our method is able to treat.

Varicose Veins

Varicose veins begin with tiny varicosities—purplish blue traces on the legs and thighs. Then, gradually, the veiny trunks become dilated, tortuous, and serpentine and develop multiple Medusa-type heads or knobs extending from the foot right up to the thigh. Varicose veins are the most obvious problems of bad circulation.

Swollen Legs

The lymphatic circulation needs equal attention. Figuratively speaking, it has the role of a sweeper, clearing away the tiny drops between the cells and generally cleaning up the body. In some people, following certain infections, for example those caused by tropical parasites such as filaria (fortunately very rare in our climate), the lymph vessels became blocked; this may also occur in certain hereditary diseases, and poor drainage of the lymphatics results. The legs swell up to an enormous size; this condition is known as elephantiasis because the legs resemble those of an elephant. A lesser degree of swelling is called edema; this is a swelling that occurs at the lower end of the limb, in the region of the ankle.

Despite their differences, the vessels in the leg have a unified circulation. This was discovered recently, when it was observed that the circulation of blood from the arteries through the vast network of tiny vessels as fine as hairs—the capillaries—which irrigate the tissues to the veins, could be short-circuited by small vessels known as shunts. The shunts pass directly from the small arteries to the veins, they are opened or closed under the influence of the central nervous system, and they control the amount of blood flowing through the capillaries.

What happens when the circulation is disturbed? The shunts, become blocked. The capillaries become inundated with blood. This blood distends the periphery and cannot flow back through the normal-sized veins. The veins therefore dilate. Their valves, which ensure the unidirectional flow of blood and prevent it from passing back down the leg, become dilated and ineffective. The intervascular tissue spaces are inundated with fluid, and the lymphatics can no longer adequately drain it away. So the entire circulatory function of the limb becomes disturbed.

Heavy Legs

We are all familiar with the symptoms of poor veinous circulation in the legs. They ache and feel heavy at the end of the day; there is a feeling of pressure, as if they have been tightened in a vise—this is particularly common among people who are on their feet all day.

Some people think that underfloor heating may also be responsible for an increase in the volume of the legs.

Swelling

Edema (that is, swelling due to accumulation of fluid) sets in gradually. Ankles that were swollen during the day but went down in the evening (especially if the feet were raised) remain permanently swollen. The edema does not disappear.

Tiny varicosities, as fine as hairs, appear—as we have already mentioned. Then larger varicosities appear, with all the ensuing complications. One of these is varicose ulcers (that is, holes in the skin that will not heal, but ooze fluid and are horribly painful). The ulcers are often accompanied by eczema of the surrounding area, and brownish stains that discolor the leg, indicating that blood that has leaked into the subcutaneous tissues has not been reabsorbed and has left its pigment behind; it is this pigment—Laemoglobin—which stains the skin. Superficial phlebitis, which is a dilation and chronic inflammation of the veins, is an additional complication; and the skin, deprived of its normal nutrition, becomes thin and shiny and shrinks, while the fluid that has seeped out of the vessels compresses them, causing the blood to stagnate and the legs to swell, so that a vicious circle results, with the blood vessels unable to perform normally their circulatory function.

Three points can be used to treat the esthetic problems of the legs, such as edema, heavy legs, varicosities, etc. These points should be stimulated regularly several times a day for two to three minutes. You should accompany massage with the exercises which we will describe later.

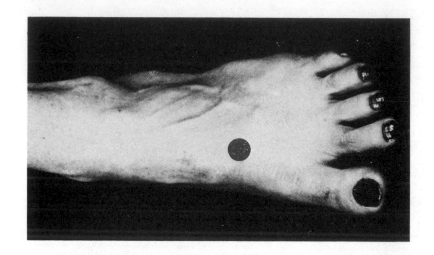

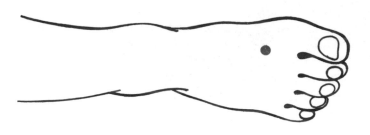

The first point is on the foot, at the
top of the space that separates the first
toe from the second, at the junction of
the two bones.

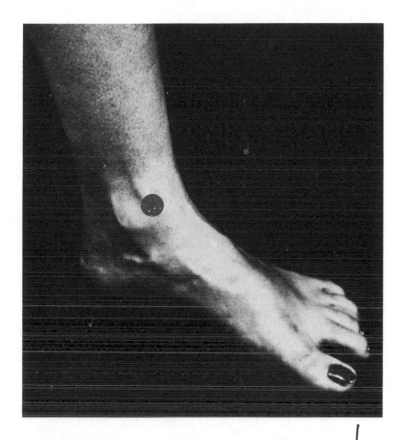

The second point is on the fold of the
dorsal crease of the foot, against the
inside of the ankle.

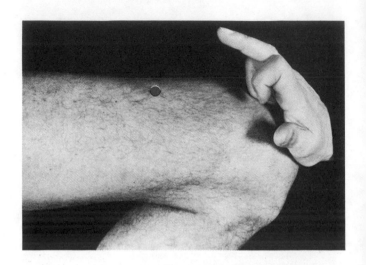

To locate the third point, place the
palm of the hand against the knee cap
while bending the knee. The top of
the middle finger will indicate the
point on the lower part of the thigh.

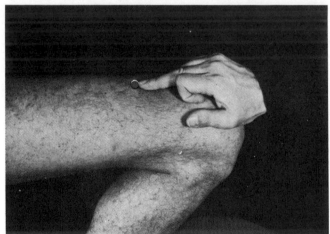

The treatment is particularly effective for tired legs—after a long day on your feet, for example.

The heart plays an essential role in arterial circulation, sending the blood out to the extremities of the body. But there is, in effect, a second heart, which returns the blood and the fluids through the veins; this is in the legs and under the foot, where a sponge full of blood, is compressed by movements and pumps the blood back to the heart: it is called the "plantar sole of Lejars," from the name of the discoverer. The calf muscles also represent a "muscular heart" for the venous blood. This is why, as with the face, the combination of movements and massage will improve the circulation of the lower limbs and enhance the appearance of the legs.

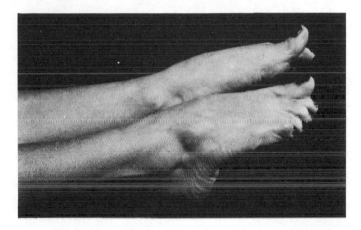

For the first movement, which is very simple, the legs should be outstretched. Flex the feet, lifting the toes sharply forward toward the legs in a quick movement; these movements drive the blood away from the extremity of the foot toward the heart.

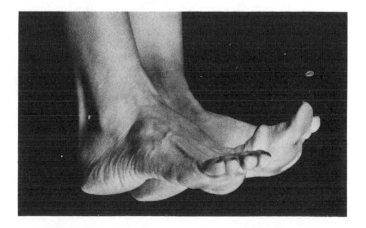

For the second movement, lie with the
legs outstretched and then draw them
in to the chest suddenly, breathing out
when they are drawn up and
breathing in as they are relaxed.

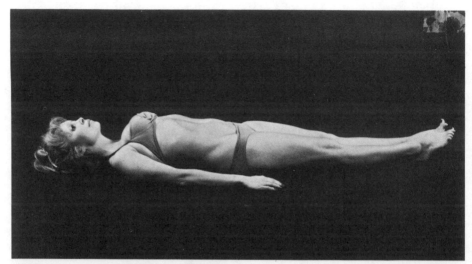

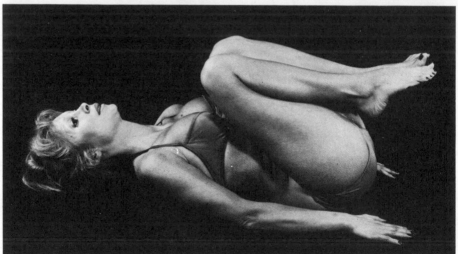

These two important movements
should be combined with stimulation
of the points already mentioned.

Safeguard the Health of Your Feet and Avoid Corns and Bunions

Our poor feet! . . . How we maltreat them! Often, of course, deformities are the results of accidents or rheumatism, but often, too, we ourselves are responsible, simply through carelessness or ignorance. Stiletto heels for example! Some women try to walk perched on four-inch-high heels, forcing their toes into the tiny closed triangular apex of the shoe, thus squashing and distorting them. Wearing such shoes over a number of years can cause irreparable damage to the feet.

The most common deformity is when the big toe is no longer straight but bends inward toward the other toes, sometimes even overlapping them. This forms on one side of the foot what is known as a hallux valgus. In like manner the little toe may also turn in—that is, both the big and the small toe are turned toward the three middle toes, squashing them or overlapping them.

But even worse can happen.

When we walk normally, particularly when barefoot, our foot rests on three points: the heel at the back, the base of the big toe at the front, and the base of the little toe at the side. These are the normal support points of the body when upright. If the foot has been badly deformed by poor fitting shoes, not only are the toes squashed and overlapping, but the sole of the front of the foot becomes rounded and, instead of two forward rest points, we have only one—in the middle of the front part of the sole.

The central part of the front of the foot was never meant to bear the weight of the body: when it has to, it can become extremely painful, and blisters, corns, and callouses appear, which in turn cause pain and stiffening. There are as many joints in the foot as there are in the hand. Instead of using them constantly, as we do the joints in the hand and fingers, thus keeping them mobile and flexible, we literally imprison our feet for the whole day. It is hardly surprising then that they become stiffened into a bad position. The muscles become stiff and spastic, and all the tiny joints rigid and ossified, as when a limb is set in plaster.

In order to prevent our feet causing serious pain once we reach middle age, certain exercises and the stimulation of specific points are essential.

First, as with the face and legs, movement of the foot is essential. Walk barefoot as often as possible. "Mobilize" your toes every evening in the following manner:

Stretch, or have someone stretch, your toes until you hear a click. Then bend and flex them as much as possible into a raised position.

Then flex the joints in the middle of the foot until you hear a similar clicking sound.

Stimulate the following points while you are completing these movements.

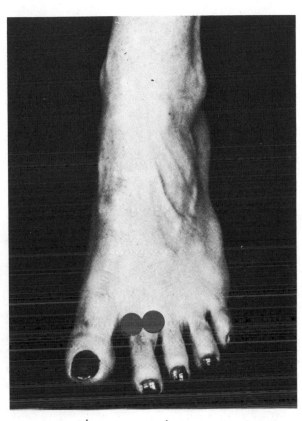

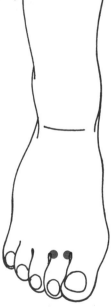

There are two points to stimulate at the base of each toe. Do this while practicing the above flexing movements. This is especially effective for the big toe.

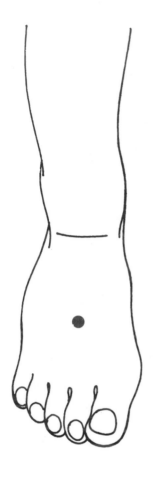

Another useful point that will help generally to ease the movements of the foot is in the very middle of the foot, halfway along and halfway across.

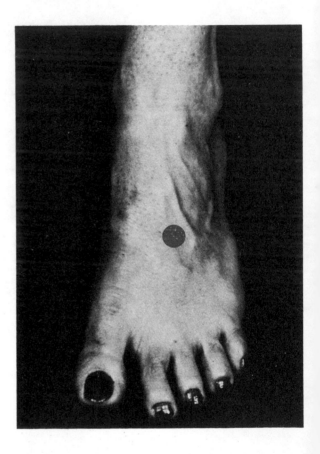

If you combine the movements with the stimulations, you will prevent deformed feet and the accompanying corns and bunions.

The Vertebral Column

How to Safeguard the Vertebral Column

The vertebral column is so important to our posture, and therefore to our general health, that anyone with the slightest trouble in this area should see a spinal specialist at least once a year—as often as we visit the dentist. Meanwhile, using a combination of stimulation of specific points and exercises, we can maintain the correct posture and balance of our vertebral column.

The Vertebral Column as a Whole
Redressing faults in the vertebral column is less a question of performing specific movements than of adopting the correct static positions. Practice these exercises twice a day, about ten times each.

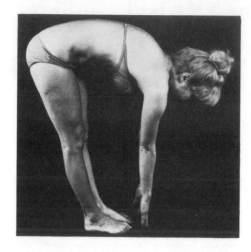

To improve sagging of the lumbar region, bend over forward and touch your toes, arching your back.

To correct forward curvature or "lordosis," stretch yourself and your limbs upward, or hang from a door jamb or chinning bar.

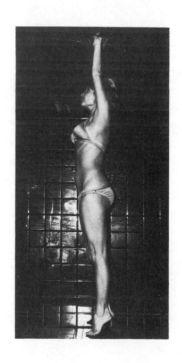

These exercises, which act on specific parts of the vertebral column, should be combined with stimulation of the following points.

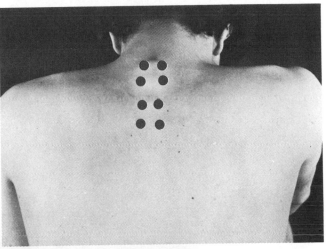

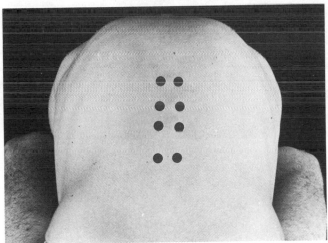

The most effective points, which have been discovered by the Chinese only recently, are situated on either side of the spine, just against it, at the bases of the bony tips of the vertebrae at all the affected levels from the nape of the neck to the middle of the back and down to the lumbar region.

Pinch the tips of the spine between two fingers, then stimulate deeply for a few minutes. You can use stimulation alone, or combine it with the exercises we have described above.

There are also effective points some distance away from the vertebral column. Reserve two or three minutes two or three times a day for stimulation. If stimulated regularly, these points will help prevent deformation of the vertebral column and painful stiffness.

The Nape of the Neck

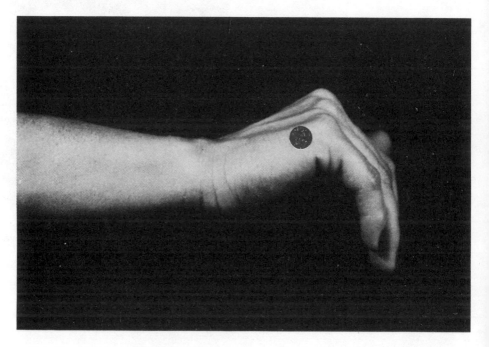

The main point is on the side of the hand along the extension of the little finger. Bend the little finger, creasing the "head line," and feel the metacarpal—the extension of the finger bone into the hand. There is a bony projection just where the bone ends, and the point is there.

The lumbar region

Two points are helpful for the lumbar region.

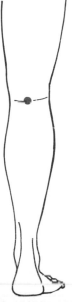

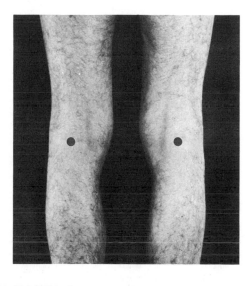

The first is at the back of the knee joint in the middle of the fold.

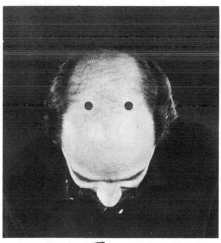

The second is on the skull, two fingers' width away from the median line on either side of the head; you will feel the junction of the two skull bones, the frontal and the parietal. The point is three fingers' width behind the hair line. Massage on the same side as the complaint.

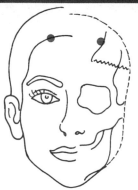

135

Conclusion

It cannot be stressed enough times that the health of the body as a whole is dependent on a healthy vertebral column. It is essential to examine vertebral joints carefully, one after the other, taking care not to neglect those that join the large bone at the bottom of the spine—the sacrum—to the large bones that form the pelvic basin. These are known as the sacroiliac joints. Deformities of the vertebral column are often caused by defects in the sacroiliac joints, particularly when the defects have not been detected in children. With age, the vertebral column begins to deform, because of tiny displacements of the minor vertebral joints that have been neglected. These displacements lead to degeneration in the joints, damage to the ligaments, and ossification, and so to the gradual deformation of the vertebral column both laterally (scoliosis) and from front to back (kyphosis). Repeated physical effort in men, during work or sport, causes pain, especially at the "hinges" or joints at the top and bottom of the column. Menopausal women often suffer from the deformity known as menopausal trophoblastic syndrome, a hump or rounded swelling immediately below the nape of the neck. When this happens the head appears to be projected beyond the dorsal column forming a convex arc and, to compensate for it, the lumbar part of the column bends forward, pushing against everything that is in front of it, including both the organs and abdominal lining. We shall consider this problem in the next chapter.

Treatment of the vertebral column demands the most scrupulous care; it is important to avoid deformities both for esthetic reasons and to prevent complications at all levels in the surrounding ligaments, muscles, and joints and in the lungs, heart, aorta, and intestines. Even the kidneys can be adversely affected and may stop functioning properly following displacement of the vertebral column.

It is therefore essential to correct abnormal posture throughout life.

The Abdominal Region
and the Stomach

How to Care for Your Abdomen and Stomach

The abdomen is usually covered by too much fat and too much skin. Excess fat is more common in men; it varies in degree from the familiar middle-age spread to an enormous pot belly. In women, the skin more often wrinkles badly and becomes slack, especially if it has been stretched by several pregnancies. Let us look at two problems; first of the underlying tissues, and second of the skin itself.

Problems of the Tissues Underneath the Skin
A protruding abdomen creates a particularly unattractive silhouette. Let us analyze the nature of such a protrusion. It has three main causes, often related to one another.

The first is due to a deformity of the vertebral column, particularly in the lumbar region—a lordosis, or forced curvature, which projects the abdomen forward. We forget all too often that we may need to correct the back before we can treat the front (see previous chapter).

The second cause is inside the abdomen: the stomach and intestines are distended with air and gas and cause the abdomen to become bloated. Such distension demands careful medical examination. Its origins need to be understood if it is to be treated properly.

However, two pressure points can relieve swelling very effectively.

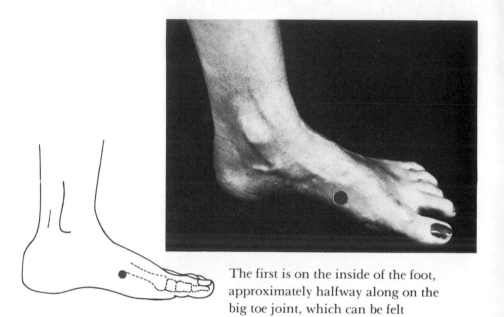

The first is on the inside of the foot, approximately halfway along on the big toe joint, which can be felt beneath the skin with your finger.

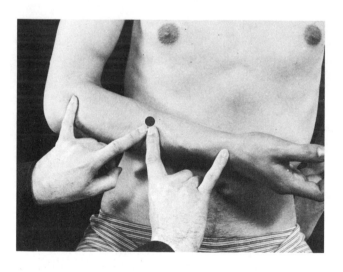

The second is on the outer edge of the forearm, halfway between the elbow and the bend of the wrist.

In the case of excessive fat, stimulation should be combined with exercises.

In order to strengthen the abdominal muscles there are several well known exercises. Here is one that does not demand any equipment.

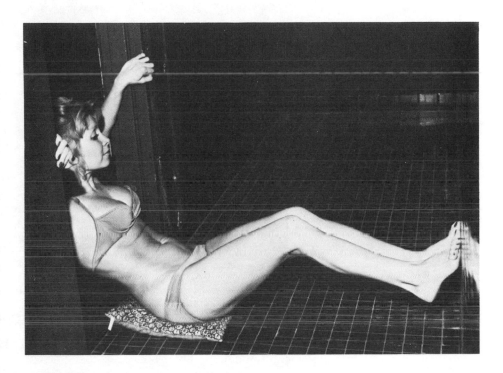

Sit down and place your hands on either side of a door frame. Press your feet against a flat stable surface or heavy weight and contract the abdomen energetically several times. This method is as effective as any to work the muscles. A dozen or so contractions once a day will maintain the tone of the abdominal muscles.

There are two useful pressure points, both of which are on the foot.
Massage these points for two or three minutes once or twice a day.

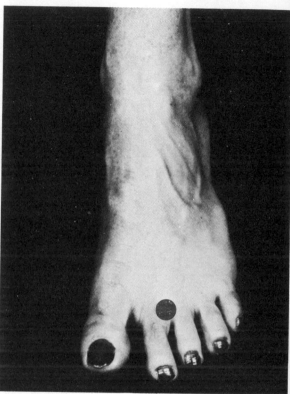

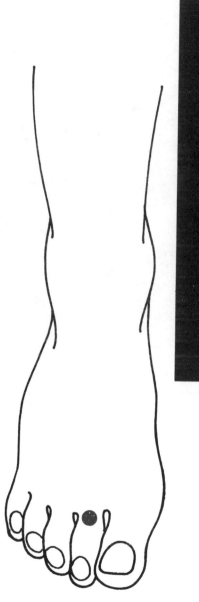

The first of these is at the base of the
second toe, on the side next to the
middle toe.

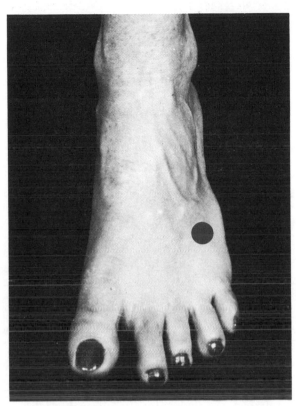

The second is in the gap between the two smallest toes, in the fourth interdigital space.

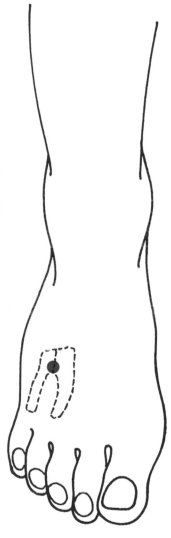

Avoiding Wrinkles and Striae of the Stomach

It is possible to treat a wrinkled or streaked stomach. The red or white streaks, or stretch marks, that appear mainly at the sides of the abdomen after the skin has been stretched for a time by abdominal distension, and then allowed to relax, are called striae. Although we tend to blame them on pregnancy or overweight, striae may also occur in thin people, and are sometimes caused by glandular or endocrine disturbances.

Two points are effective for toning up the abdomen and for treating striae. Massage these points regularly for about five minutes two or three times a day.

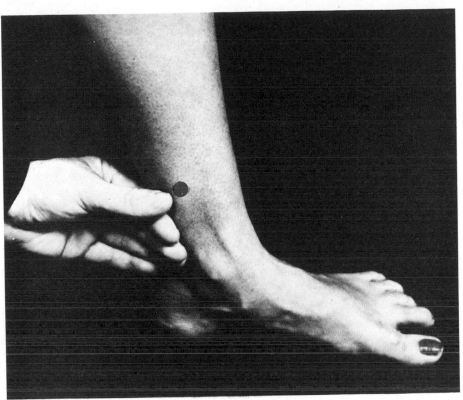

The first is an important gynecological point. It is on the inside of the leg, at the back of the tibia, one hand's width above the inner protrusion of the ankle joint, in a small hollow.

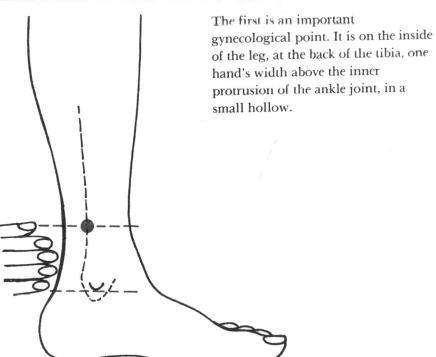

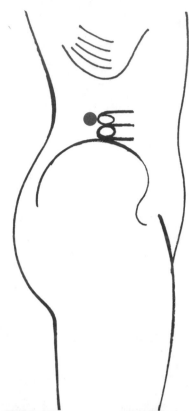

The second is above the iliac crest on the median body line, two fingers' width above the top of the crest.

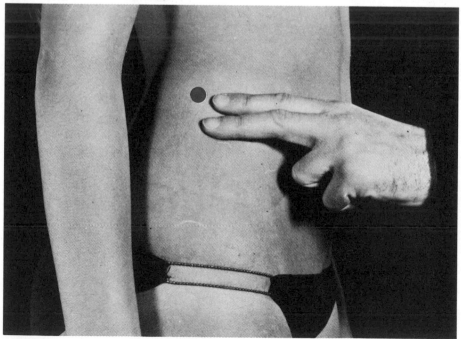

Height and Weight

How to Affect Your Height

What growing child hasn't stood in front of the mirror and said to him/herself, "If only I could grow a few inches taller!"

Vanity is not the only problem here, since growing troubles may have a number of causes, some of which science is unable to remedy. Dwarfs, for example, have an inherited glandular disease that cannot be treated.

In other cases, stunted growth is caused by a serious breakdown in the bodily functions. A child may be prevented from growing by heart or kidney disease, by certain infections, rheumatism or malnutrition.

Fortunately, however, when a child is small for his age, it is usually a question of late development, as though the growth clock had somehow temporarily slowed down or stopped. In such cases, massage of pressure points may be very effective.

On the other hand, we may occasionally want to stop our children growing into giants.

The same points are used in both cases. The Chinese points can work on the same bodily function in directly opposite ways, normalizing and regularizing the function.

Two points act in the same way. Stimulate them every day to alter the rate of growth in the direction desired. Of course, you may wish to try other methods meanwhile, but these points will help.

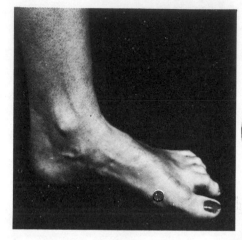

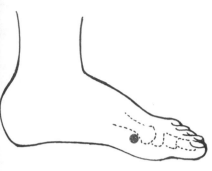

The first is under the big toe, a little behind the joint that attaches it to the foot.

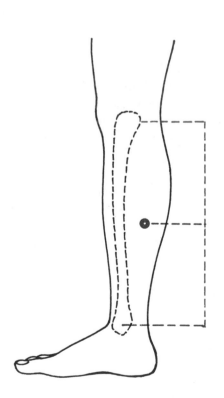

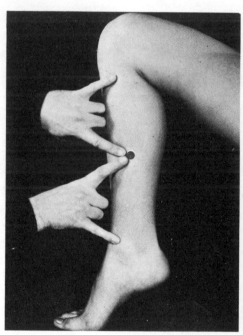

The second point is halfway up the inside of the calf.

How to Control Your Weight

One of the most widespread obsessions of western men and women is with their weight and, above all, with being overweight. Obesity is a neurosis of our age. We have put on an extra pound, we are too fat, and we become upset and despairing. This may be a long-standing problem, but there is also the temporary or labile obesity, which comes and goes. The most common form of this is the swelling in women which often occurs just before a period and is known as the premenstrual syndrome. This is due to the retention of water in the body, influenced by the female hormones, and sometimes it does not go down as soon as one hopes.

Let us look at the effective points for this complaint. Stimulating them will help you to lose weight by diuresis, that is, by the urinary elimination of the excess fluid.

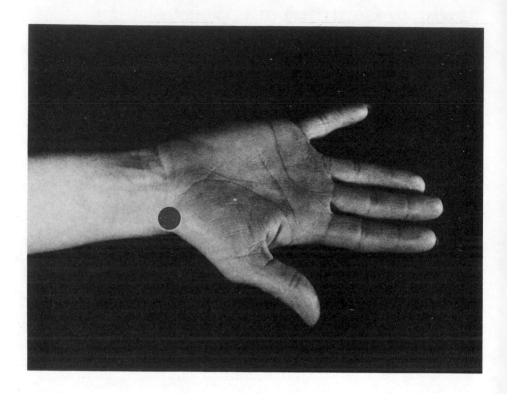

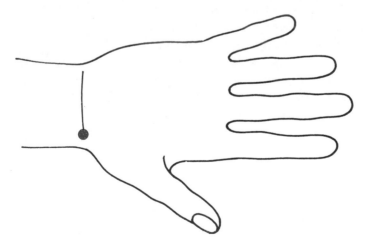

The first is on the outer side of the
wrist in the groove of the pulse.

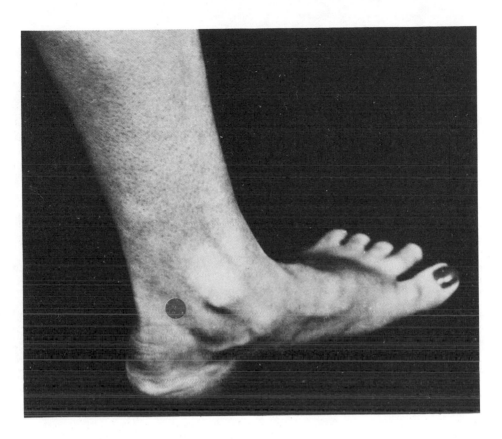

The second point is on the inside of the foot behind the ankle bone, in the middle of the upper edge of the bone right at the back of the foot.

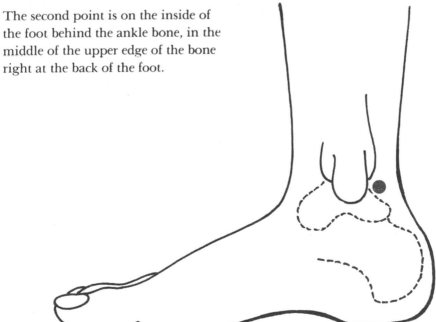

How to Control Obesity

Gross and prolonged obesity is an enormous problem. Acupuncture is just one of many ways of helping people who are seriously overweight, and it can be very effective as an easy, convenient, and natural form of treatment.

Obesity is not just physically undesirable. It may be in itself a serious form of illness. It can cause varicose veins and leg ulcers, afflictions of the joints of the vertebral column and the legs, degeneration of the knee joints, ankles, and feet; but, above all it may lead to complications in the circulatory system, the heart and blood vessels. Cardiac accidents, coronary thrombosis or cerebral vascular accidents—"strokes" with paralysis—are more common in the obese than in normal people.

There is a relation between mortality rate and obesity. As we put on extra pounds, so our life expectancy decreases. American life insurance companies have calculated the risks in this area and now demand supplementary premium payments from people carrying excess weight.

Considerable progress has been made in recent years in discovering the origins of obesity. It is often hereditary; from birth the child is often fatter than normal, and this obesity is often associated with diabetes in later life. Obesity may also be the result of poor eating habits. A child who has always been overfed will tend to overeat all his life and remain fat.

Obesity can also have psychological causes. It may be triggered off by distress, anguish, or even boredom. It is very common for people who are upset or bored to nibble constantly and to find comfort by helping themselves to everything in the refrigerator that they can lay their hands on.

Obesity may also be glandular, or it can cause glandular disorders, which in women may lead to cessation of menstruation and even to sterility. The contraceptive pill has often been accused of causing weight gain—sometimes justifiably, although here the cause is usually fluid retention.

Obese people fall into two physical types:
—Androids, or the masculine type; here the shoulders are wider than the pelvis.
—Gynaecoids, or the feminine type; these people have huge buttocks and a "stomach apron"—a pendulous overlapping layer of abdominal fat that hangs down in front of them.

Whichever type you are, being overweight is a problem that must be dealt with.

There is an ever expanding industry in slimming foods and medicines, yet one seems to be more dangerous than another, causing water or muscle loss rather than making the fat disappear.

Similarly, in the case of appetite depressants the nervous system is stimulated, and the side effects are often far more serious than the initial weight problem. A change in diet is the only sensible answer.

There are several kinds of diet. We shall not discuss these, but there are some pressure points that can be of help in obesity since they may aid depression of the appetite.

There are three points.

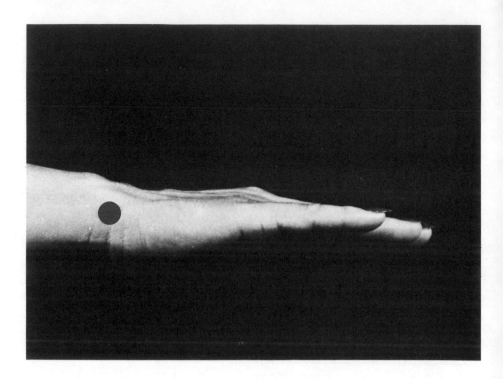

The first is on the inner edge of the
bend of the wrist, on the small
pointed bone called the pisiform. This
is just where the hand joins the wrist
on the little finger side.

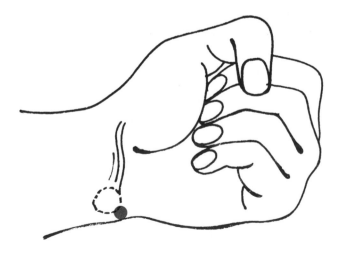

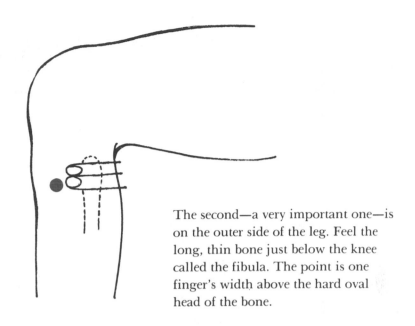

The second—a very important one—is on the outer side of the leg. Feel the long, thin bone just below the knee called the fibula. The point is one finger's width above the hard oval head of the bone.

This point has a general effect on the whole body. Stimulate it regularly two or three times every day for about five minutes.

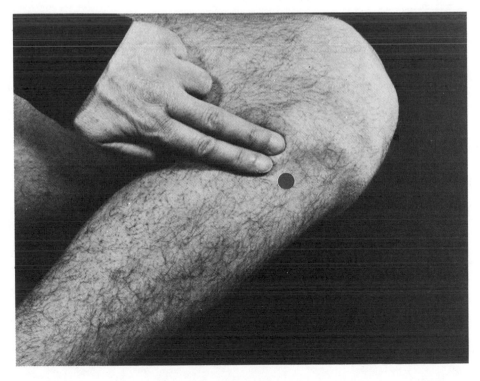

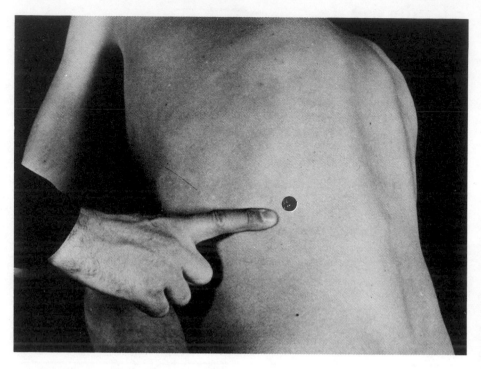

The third point is on the back at the
tip of the bottom rib. Stimulate it
several times a day.

These points are highly effective in
aiding weight loss.

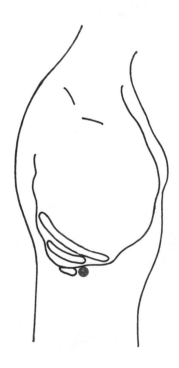

Underweight

Obesity is not the only weight problem, however. Being underweight, though not so serious, is also best avoided. First we need to know why the person is underweight. Weight loss may occur when the patient is ill, or after a pregnancy (although the new mother is usually overweight). There is also a constitutional thinness, a body build known as the asthenie—the subject is thin, but in no way adversely affected by it. However, being excessively underweight is physically unattractive. Nobody wants to look like a walking skeleton.

So it is useful to know the point that will allow you to gain a few pounds. Stimulate it every day. Your absorption of food will improve, and you will gain weight.

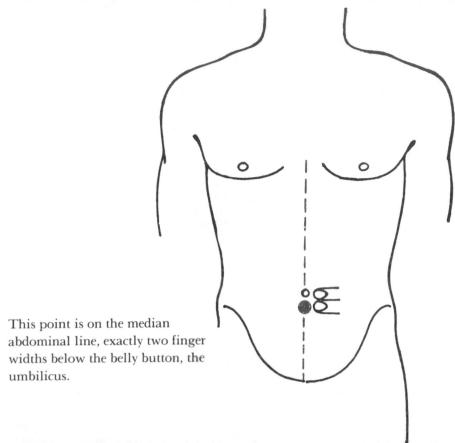

This point is on the median abdominal line, exactly two finger widths below the belly button, the umbilicus.

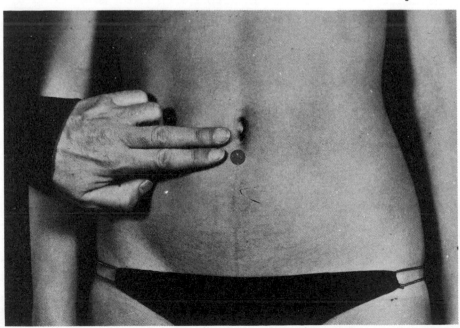

Skin Care

Introduction to Skin Care

The skin, the envelope that covers our entire body, is the tissue through which acupuncture acts.

There is a great number of skin diseases. We have already dealt with some of these afflictions in our chapters on the face and abdomen, but it is not within the scope of this book to present a treatise on dermatology. We shall merely look at the way in which pressure points can relieve unpleasant skin defects.

Prevent and treat spots and rashes

Vitiligo

As we saw when studying the face, the skin can become affected with black, gray, or brown spots. Sometimes, however, there are patches of skin that are too white and milky: these are depigmentation spots, or *vitiligo*. They have no known origin, or etiology; and there is no known treatment for them, strictly speaking. This is why you need to use a very precise acupressure point which, if stimulated regularly, may bring relief.

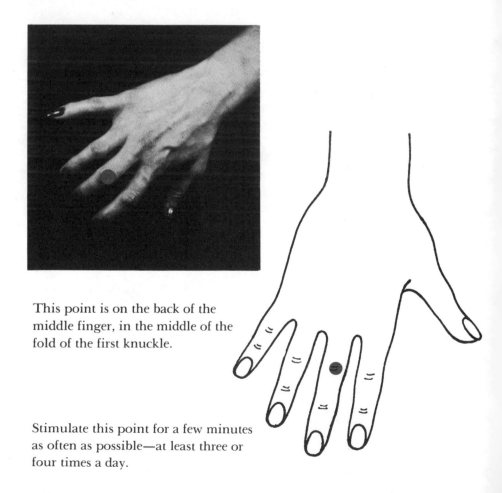

This point is on the back of the middle finger, in the middle of the fold of the first knuckle.

Stimulate this point for a few minutes as often as possible—at least three or four times a day.

164

Rashes and Red Flushes

Unlike *vitiligo,* rashes cover areas of the body with red patches or spots. Rashes may be symptomatic, harmless and temporary, as in the illnesses that affect young children, such as measles. But they may also be caused by allergic reactions, and can be temporary, as with urticaria, or chronic and almost permanent, as with the unfortunate condition of eczema, where the skin constantly peels, weeps, and suppurates. However, we shall not be looking at problems within the province of general medicine here.

Psoriasis occurs first in the form of red, crater-like spots that later become gray and scaly, and that may cover the entire body and cause the sufferer considerable social embarrassment.

Psoriasis needs continuous medical care. But two points may help to reduce its intensity and prevent the condition from deteriorating. Stimulate them energetically for two or three minutes every morning and evening.

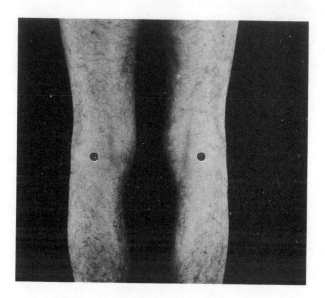

The first is the major point for all skin infections. It is at the back of the knee in the middle of the fold.

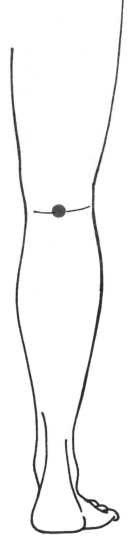

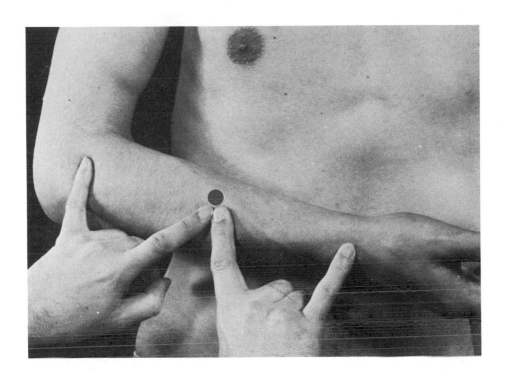

The second is in the middle of the outer surface of the forearm, where the two axes intersect, as shown in the diagram.

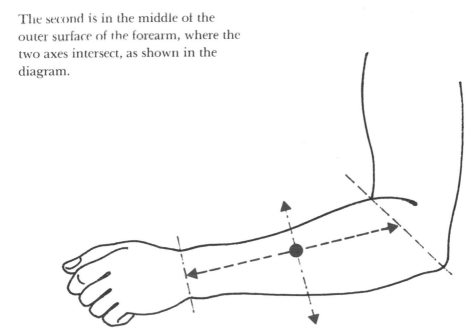

Treating Warts and Growths

Another annoying complaint that can affect the skin manifests itself in the form of tiny abnormal swellings or growths of different sorts: these are tumors. Do not let the word tumor, which in most people's minds is synonymous with cancer, mislead you. We are dealing here with tiny benign tumors that distort the skin and give it a grubby, unpleasant appearance.

We shall consider two sorts of tumor that our therapy can help. First warts, and second molluscums—small outgrowths on tiny stalks that hang on the skin.

Everyone is familiar with warts. They come in different forms. The common or "vulgar" warts can grow anywhere on the body, and particularly on the hands and fingers, where they appear as small raised scabs covered with tiny spots.

The most painful form of wart is the plantar wart, or verruca, which grows in the skin on the underside of the foot. It can impede walking to such a degree that it is sometimes wrongly diagnosed as rheumatism. Surgical treatment of verrucas is often unsatisfactory, particularly as the surgery involved may be more damaging to the body than the initial complaint. If part of the verruca is left behind, it will grow back, and, if too much tissue is removed, the wounded foot may develop an ulcer; walking is very painful and difficult, and the healing process may be very slow.

Flat warts on the back of the hand are equally unpleasant, and can cause the sufferer considerable embarrassment.

Finally, venereal warts may appear in the genital area. These are cauliflower-like in shape, they are extremely unpleasant, and may smell very bad. They are also contagious.

Molluscums and verrucas are also caused by contagious viral infections. We can be infected in humid places such as at swimming pools. Such infections need a certain environment in order to develop. Thanks to acupressure, we are able to act on that environment. Stimulate these points vigorously for two or three minutes several times a day.

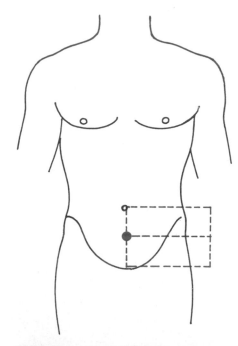

The first point is on the abdomen, halfway between the naval and the pubic region, in the median line.

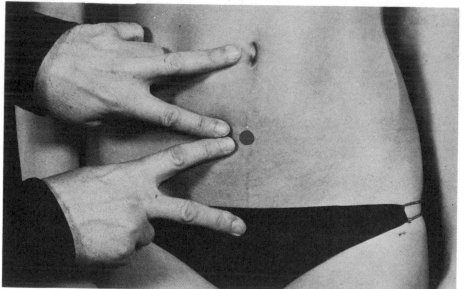

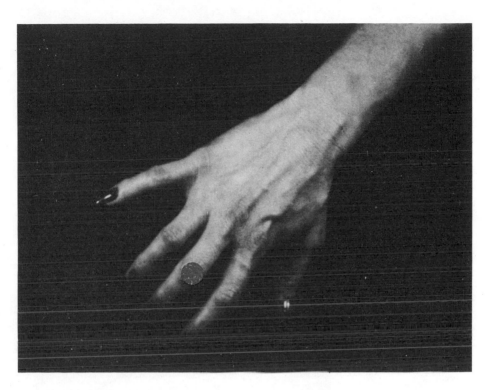

The second point is on the middle finger, on the knuckle between the first and second phalanges.

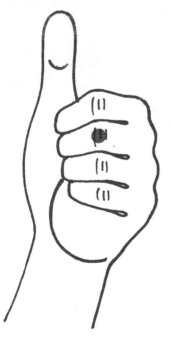

There are two more points to mention.

The first, which concerns hand warts, is on the outside of the forearm, four fingers' width below the point of the elbow.

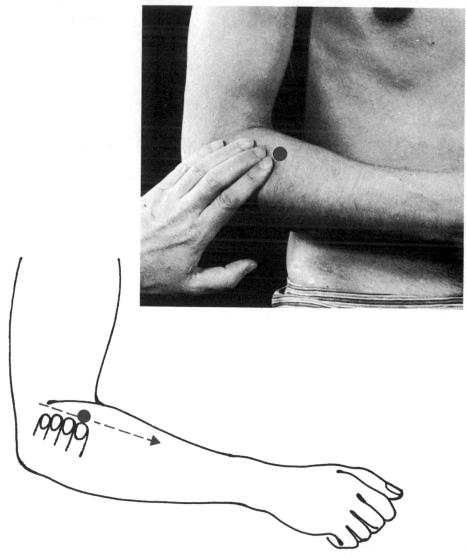

The second, which concerns the legs, is on the outer side of the legs, two fingers' width above the middle of the line joining the knee to the ankle, a little beyond the bone and right in the middle of the muscle mass.

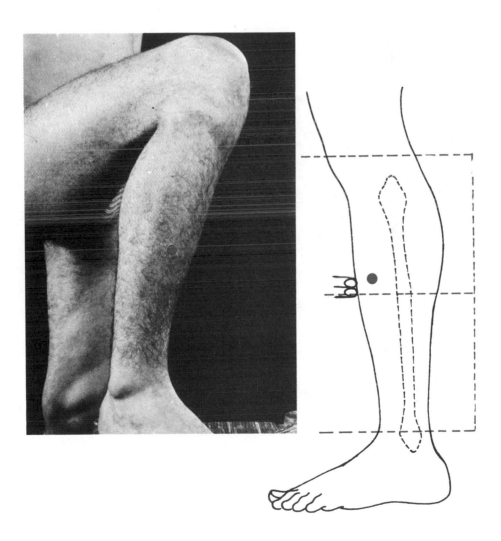

Avoid and Treat Chilblains

Although chilblains are only temporary and are not too distressing to look at, they are very painful. Circulatory disturbance at the extremities results in malnutrition of the skin, which causes chapped splits and sores of the fingers and toes.

One point is very effective.

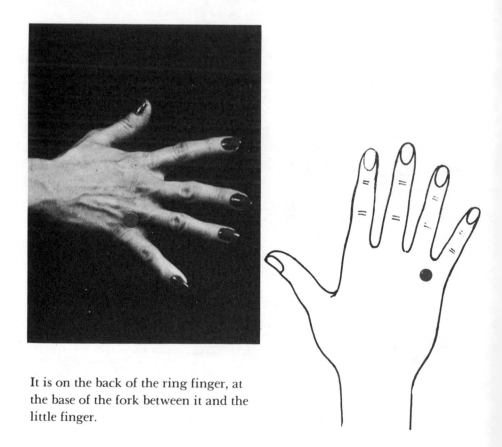

It is on the back of the ring finger, at the base of the fork between it and the little finger.

Prevent and Treat Superfluous Hair

Women normally find superfluous hair such as traces of a moustache, or hairs on the breasts or abdomen, undesirable.

Hairs on the abdomen are typical of the masculine pattern of growth of pubic hairs, whereas the feminine pubic growth is flat-topped and triangular.

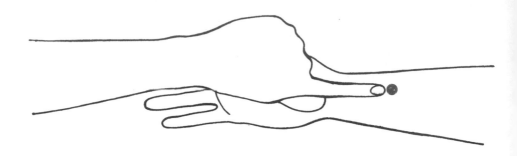

The point that is effective for excess
hair is the same as the one for acne. It
is on the inside of the wrist.

Lock the hands, as we described for
acne, and the first index finger will
indicate the point, as shown in the
photograph.

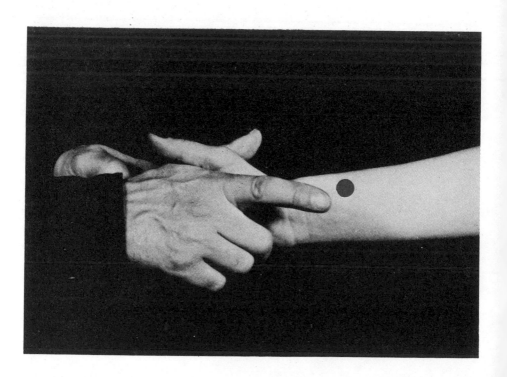

From the Past . . . to the Future

The use of acupuncture is now so widespread in the West that most of the theories that attempt to provide an explanation for its action are well known.

We shall merely summarize them here briefly, and then go on to discuss the important recent discoveries made in China and the West that throw light on the way in which acupuncture produces its effect. We shall also describe new methods of stimulation.

Acupuncture goes back a long time. The Chinese are not able to pinpoint the origins precisely for the following reason: approximately 500 B.C. the Chinese Emperor Hoang-Ti ordered the destruction of all writings and documents that had existed before his accession to power. Everything had to be subordinated to him, from agriculture to moral precepts, and from medicine to the famous Great Wall, which he had built. After his death, the few remaining sages who survived him had to reproduce all the destroyed texts from memory and could not avoid omissions, repetitions, and error. Acupuncture certainly existed before this tyrannical emperor. Gold and silver needles have been found in the tombs of princes and princesses who lived 1500 years B.C.

We shall never discover the exact origins of acupuncture; it would be fascinating to trace its very beginnings, the first gropings toward a method of treatment, the initial failures leading to the successes of the scrupulously careful Chinese observers.

However, from the documents that we do possess, we know that acupuncture dates back over twenty centuries, and its underlying principles have remained intact and have been strengthened by their incorporation into the Chinese philosophical tradition. Let us look at those fundamental principles.

For the Chinese, the universe is a whole, in which—as Einstein was to show many centuries later—matter and energy are two aspects of a single reality. This vital force—the Tao—is diffused throughout the entire cosmos of which each one of us is a tiny part in constant communication with the whole. The Tao manifests itself in two ways, or, more exactly, as two different aspects of the same truth: these two elements are called Yin and Yang. Yin and Yang complement one another and merge without disturbing each other; they do this as inevitably as day follows night or ice becomes water.

Human beings are bathed in this energy whose sources, both external and internal, are numerous: the air we breathe, the food we eat and the psychological force and the sexual energy that emanate from us. The Tao permeates our entire body and every centimeter of our skin. There is a continuous flow of vital energy along special lines or channels just under the surface of the body that correspond with the major organs. In the West we call these lines "meridians." If energy stops flowing, in other words if there is an obstruction somewhere along one of these meridians, illness will develop. Along these meridians there are acupuncture points that allow the flow of energy to be modified both qualitatively and quantitatively.

Thus massage of the carefully and specifically chosen points allows the normal flow of energy to re-establish itself and, as a result, good health returns.

Tradition has taught us which points to puncture to "tone" or stimulate the corresponding organs, and, conversely, which points to use to "disperse," that is calm them.

When this strange medicine was introduced to the West, it produced cries of shock and outrage, since it shook the foundations on which Western medicine rested. It took considerable courage for doctors in the West to adopt Chinese methods of treatment, as they did between about 1930 and 1960. However, they were encouraged by the effectiveness of the methods and by the excellent results they obtained and by the enthusiasm, which was sometimes excessive, of their patients. And yet in established circles hostility and antagonism remained, and the practitioners of acupuncture continued to be dismissed as charlatans and confidence tricksters.

But gradually some remarkable evidence came out of China: doctors in the West were astonished to find themselves watching the amazing sight of surgery being performed without conventional anesthesia on a patient in whom analgesia, that is absence of pain, was achieved simply by inserting a needle into a specific point in the body. It was equally astounding to see proof of the treatment of congenital deafness, which Western medicine had failed to cure. A succession of films, televised sequences, study visits, reports and documents, brought irrefutable evidence to the West.

Slowly the wall of incomprehension and hostility began to crumble; and finally it became possible to study the method in detail, in an attempt to penetrate its secrets, to understand its working mechanisms, and to improve still more their effectiveness.

In China doctors made an enormous effort to adopt Western methods, and to adapt them where necessary to complement their own. It was felt to be important to build a bridge between modern Western science and the traditional Chinese. Chang-Hsiang-tung of the Institute of Physiology in Shanghai wrote recently: "Every Western doctor who came to visit us reacted differently to our medicine. Some would look upon it sceptically and would dismiss it because it lacked a scientific explanation. Others on the contrary, were blindly devoted to it, and refused to hear of the tiniest variation to the ancient dogma. Both these attitudes are wrong." And, we might add, "The truth is halfway between the two."

The traditional teaching provides us with a wealth of observations, facts, and techniques of use. But we are in no way showing lack of respect if we wish to find a scientific explanation for acupuncture to satisfy our curiosity, to allow us to perfect the method, and to deepen our knowledge of the physiology of our bodies.

Research work was undertaken both in China and the West, in particular in France, Sweden, the United States, and Canada, which brought impressive results in a remarkably short time, results that have taken their place among the most highly sophisticated research of our time.

We have discussed the main body of these results, explaining to a large degree how acupuncture works, in the earlier book, *How to Give Yourself Relief from Pain by the Simple Pressure of a Finger*, and we recommend the reader to refer to it.

Here we shall give a resumé of what was said before, concentrating more specifically on the discoveries that have been published within the last years.

The Skin . . . and What Lies Beneath It

1 It has been known for a long time that the acupuncture points and meridians at skin level possess particular properties. Pain sensitivity—which this book will teach you to discover when you locate the points—is greater for the patient, and electrical sensation is felt more intensely by him, at these points than in adjacent areas. Doctors have spent years using ingenious apparatus to record electrical currents and resistance at the acupuncture points and meridians lines and comparing them with other parts of the skin. However, the smallest amount of pressure on the skin will alter resistance and this of course includes the pressure exerted by the recording electrodes themselves, so the use of these methods has been rejected. Nonetheless, these researches have been the starting point of new hypotheses—all related to the discovery that there is an alternative nervous system at skin level.

2 What exactly is there under the skin? What are these receptors which obey the stimulation of tiny needles or the pressure of our fingers and transmit their beneficial orders to the innermost regions of the body? What are their properties? What is their nature? Are they all alike, or do some differ from others? Until very recently, there have been no answers to these questions. However, a series of Chinese research teams at the universities of Shanghai and Shensi, the medical college at Anhui and the Xian team have made exciting discoveries using advanced methods. There are hundreds of receptors, and there appear to be at least 500 different varieties, according to the latest findings. The majority of them are in the muscles.

As we know, muscles are made up of many bundles of parallel fibers. The acupuncture receptors have been located in the deepest fibers—in other words, in the very heart of the muscle. It is extraordinary that they remain sensitive even when the muscle is paralyzed with a known poison—curare (the famous American Indian arrow poison)—or following an illness or accident.

There are other receptors in the muscle tendons (what are sometimes referred to in everyday language as "guides," or "meat nerves," although they are not in fact nerves at all), and yet more in the joints and the skin. Curiously, receptors are also incorporated into the nervous system, for example in the motor disc of the muscle, which triggers off contraction, and in the feeling corpuscles. Some are even at the extremities of exposed nerve endings. And yet, when pressure is applied to these points, they all transmit a particular sensation, the special feeling that you will have become familiar with in using this book. It is very difficult to describe—the closest we can get is to call it a sort of bruising or distension, quite unlike the normal sensation of pain.

This is not surprising. Extending their investigations, Chinese researchers have shown that the nerve fibers that transmit the two sorts of sensation are in fact different. These fibers are numbered according to their diameter from 1 to 4. While 2 and 3 transmit all sorts of sensation simultaneously, the 4 fibers transmit only the sensation particular to acupuncture. The task of isolating these fibers and determining their routes and connections is an immense one, which remains to be undertaken.

But there is more: two other phenomena have been discovered by Chinese scientists.

The first is that the points are in some way specialized according to their topography. In other words, one point will act on the skin, another on the stomach, yet another on the nervous system, and this is determined by the area of the body they correspond with.

Secondly, Chinese researchers have discovered very recently that a sensation is exchanged between the subject being treated (whether by needles or finger pressure) and the operator. This "finger sensation," as it is called, manifests itself in a feeling of heavyness and contraction at the end of the operator's finger.

It would seem then, if these discoveries are confirmed, that there is an exchange of energy between the operator and the patient. This opens up innumerable questions about the relationship between subjects and the exchanges between the internal and external energies. These issues are very close to traditional Chinese ideas and open doors on to fascinating avenues for the future.

Let us now look at how stimulation acts at the different levels of the nervous system.

3   *At spinal cord level:* The increasing use of acupuncture to replace chemical anesthesia has allowed us to confirm the "gate control theory" of pain which was described in some detail in *How to Give Yourself Relief from Pain by the Simple Pressure of a Finger* and is summarized here briefly.

The stimulation of the group 4 fibers blocks the impulses transmitted by the other fibers and prevents their passage to the part of the brain where they are identified as painful sensations. Metaphorically speaking, the gate is shut on pain. This, in part, explains how surgical operations can be performed using acupuncture instead of conventional anesthesia, and how, as I have shown in my previous book, acupuncture can relieve a variety of everyday aches and pains. Recent research has thrown more light onto these ideas.

It seems that the "gate" does not exist at only one level of the spinal cord, and that the length of the spinal cord and the number of segments brought into play depends on the intensity and amount of stimulation. Let us look at an example.

The point identified for curing acne on the face, when pressed lightly, will act effectively on the facial skin; if it is stimulated more energetically, it will act on aches in the face; if it is stimulated with a needle or electrically, it will allow us to perform surgery painlessly in this region. At this stage we will be aware of the diffusion of this action to other areas of the body (the neck and shoulder, in this particular case), since the more intense the stimulation, the greater the number of segments of the spinal cord affected, which in turn affect the regions of the body that correspond with them. This explains why points in the arms usually act on the upper part of the body, the head, and the neck, while points on the legs affect the lower parts, the back, and stomach. As stimulation becomes more intense, so other areas of the body become affected. This is why several different points can treat the same complaint. It will all depend on the nature and intensity of stimulation.

The triggering off of these different stages is not merely electrical. It seems likely that chemical substances known as mediators are released, and we shall consider these next.

4   *Brain level:* Here is one of the most fascinating findings of recent research. Professor Guillemin of the University of California at La Jolla, a Nobel Prize winner for medicine, has discovered that "hard" drugs, especially morphine, are only able to act because substances very similar to opium derivatives are secreted by the brain. These varieties of natural morphine are released by acupuncture. It has been demonstrated in China, and in Canada by Professor Pomeranz of the University of Toronto, that, after stimulation with needles, the cerebro-spinal fluid that bathes the brain contains increased quantities of natural morphines. Similar results have been observed when cross sections of rat brains are examined immediately after acupuncture.

There is proof, then, that stimulation of acupuncture points brings about changes at the highest levels in the workings of the central nervous system. Here again, science has made progress recently.

As we have said, different sorts of natural morphines have been discovered which may be divided into two main groups: encephalins and endorphines. Members of the first group are secreted into the brain and nearby glands, especially the hypophysis. They play a normal role in this area. But they are not exclusively linked to any specific area. According to the need and the intensity of stimulation

182

they can spread deeper and deeper into the various areas of brain tissue. From a simple trickle or stream, they can become a river in flood. So once again we come back to the distinction between moderate stimulation, which creates a localized reaction, and more intense action, which triggers off a more diffuse influence. We can thus appreciate the magnificent range of effects at the acupuncturist's fingertips, which will allow him to bring relief to an ache or to treat a far more serious and widespread complaint. What is more, we are beginning to understand how, outside the nervous system itself, the method may act on the entire body.

5 *Action on the body as a whole:* For a long time experiments have shown that acupuncture acts on the major body organs—the heart, the lungs, and the digestive system—in a way that cannot be explained through the nervous system alone. For example, how can we explain that stimulation of a certain point triggers off an increase in the number of red blood corpuscles in the blood, while a different point can cause an increase in the number of white corpuscles?

The explanation partly lies with the second variety of natural morphines, the endorphines. These substances are secreted by the nervous system and are to be found in more or less all parts of the body, where they regulate the life of our cells. Further explanation is called for here. We know that the body is made up of a great number of cells juxtaposed with each other. Each one has a specific role in its area, but each one receives its orders either through the intermediary of the nervous system or, less directly, through the intermediary of hormones. We know that these are chemical messengers that enter the blood via the glands—among the most important of which are the thyroid, the ovary, the pancreas, and the testicle. These chemical messengers come from opposite ends of the body to instruct the cells: "get rid of your fat," says the thyroid hormone; "Expel your sugar," says insulin from the pancreas. But most of these hormones do not actually enter the cell, they only knock against the protective cell wall.

There must, therefore, be a second substance that triggers off the chemical mechanism inside the cell so that the hormonal order is carried out. How, this second substance, or "second chemical messenger" as its discoverer Professor Sutherland has named it, is almost unique. It is called by a rather forbidding name that is usually shortened to Cyclic AMP. It is as though there is an intelligence standing on the doorstep of the cell like a good housekeeper crying out when there is a knock on the door, "Here's the postman."

Since we know that no chemical molecule exists with an intelligence of its own, there must be informers in the cell wall that alter the response according to need. These are the endorphines, which are liberated by acupuncture and which organize a beneficial response to the disturbances of the affected areas.

The existence of regulators or organizers at all levels gives us a glimpse of the enormous complexity of the use of acupuncture, whose workings remain to be fully investigated in the centuries to follow. We are no longer dealing with a series of chemical chain reactions, as in the case of the manufacture of sugar or the breaking down of fats, which the chemist can undertake in his laboratory. We are talking about infinitely more complex functions, which indicate the existence of an organizing principle, a computer, we might say, controlling the equilibrium of the body. And it is on this computer that our points act, calming it here and exciting it there and, what is even better, we can alter the effect according to the place and intensity of stimulation.

We can put the internal energies of the body in contact and harmony with the energies of the environment, and achieve the vital equilibrium, the condition of perfect well-being.

Is this not the finest reward for the oldest medicine in the world, to see it become one of the newest and most promising for the future?

And does this not provide the best justification for the use of the points we have described, to safeguard our health and beauty?

Conclusion

One of the essential aims of every human being should be to look after his or her body.

As we said at the beginning of the book: beauty equals health; hence the necessity, it seemed to us, for a book dealing with beauty care. We are particularly anxious to discourage the exclusive use of chemical products, which, whether taken internally or externally, can be harmful and dangerous. The stimulation of specific pressure points, although it is not the only effective treatment for the complaints that may afflict us, is a useful complement to other treatment, frequently very effective and never harmful.

If this book can convert a few people and lead them to use the method regularly, we shall have achieved our purpose. But our aim has been even more ambitious.

The regular use of this method has convinced us that it has an important preventive role. We feel we have performed an important service if we have managed to communicate an effective means of safeguarding health.

Index

Skin care, 163-76
Stiletto heels, 125
Striae on stomach, 144
Sub-labial dimple, 56
Superfluous hair, 28, 175-76

Tao, 178
Telogene phase of hair growth, 68
Thought wrinkles, 40
Thyroid gland, 81
Tonsilitis, 81
"Toothless wrinkle," 57
Tuberculoid acne, 19

Ulcers
    of skin, 119
    of leg, 154
Umbilication of nipple, 102
Underweight, 159-60

Varicose veins, 118, 119, 154
Venereal warts, 169
Venous circulation, 117

poor, symptoms of, 117-18
Verruca (plantar wart), 168
Vertebral column, 81
Vitiligo, 27, 164

Warts, 168-73
Weight
    control, during menstruation, 151-53
    loss, by diuresis, 151
    See also Obesity; Underweight
Wrinkles, 17, 38-63, 144-46
    on abdomen, 144-46
    adventurers', 42
    on cheeks, 49
    crow's feet, 63
    around eye, 58-63
    on forehead, 40-41
    around mouth and eyes, 53-57
    muscles underlying, 38
    on neck, 81
    near nose, 45
    on shoulders and arms, 84
    "toothless," 57